ZERO POINT ONE SIX

Living in Extra Time

MICK DOYLE

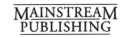
MAINSTREAM
PUBLISHING

EDINBURGH AND LONDON

Copyright © Mick Doyle, 2001
All rights reserved
The moral right of the author has been asserted

First published in Great Britain in 2001 by
MAINSTREAM PUBLISHING COMPANY (EDINBURGH) LTD
7 Albany Street
Edinburgh EH1 3UG

ISBN 1 84018 485 X

No part of this book may be reproduced or transmitted in any form
or by any means without written permission from the publisher,
except by a reviewer who wishes to quote brief passages in connection
with a review written for insertion in a newspaper, magazine or broadcast

A catalogue record for this book is available from the British Library

All photographs © the author

Typeset in Civet and Janson Text
Printed and bound in Great Britain
by Mackays of Chatham

Contents

LIVING IN EXTRA TIME

The Future is Our Own

Somewhere, along life's complacent monotone,
The sudden, frightening horror struck mercilessly,
     without apology,
Utterly changing everything with quite bewildering
     rapidity;
Later, as the cul-de-sac of a much altered way of life
Surprisingly led on to more benevolent byroads,
The new way, almost unbelievably, became enjoyable
     as before
And life worth living again.

Mick Doyle
June 2001

This book is dedicated to my wife and my
four children, my good friends, to all those who want to
make it and to those who wish to help them.

Mick Doyle

foreword

In 1985, after Ireland beat England in the Triple Crown decider at Lansdowne Road, a poster proclaimed 'DR DOYLE BRAIN TRANSPLANT SURGEON'. This was a riposte by Irish supporters to English journalists, who earlier in the year had ridiculed Mick Doyle's claims that Ireland could play running rugby, stating that such an achievement could be realised only if Irish rugby underwent a 'brain transplant'. It was somewhat ironic that ten years later Mick would sustain a potentially fatal brain injury.

Stroke is an interruption of the blood supply to the brain due to blockage of an artery or a bleed from a ruptured blood vessel (haemorrhage). The resulting brain injury may result in damage or substantial disability in survivors. 'Stroke' is essentially a lay expression. The medical terms include 'cerebrovascular accident' or 'apoplexy', but neither of these describe the dramatic nature of an individual being 'struck down'.

Because of limited knowledge about the condition, stroke is associated with many myths and misconceptions. There is a widespread belief that nothing can be done, and patients and carers often become profoundly depressed. Research, however, has revealed that rehabilitation has a major part to play in improving

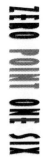

11

their outcome. Accordingly, this contribution from a high-profile individual such as Mick Doyle, who sustained a stroke due to a haemorrhage, is most welcome. It charts his progress from coma, with its very poor prognosis, to improving mobility and physical recovery. He identifies the importance of his own commitment and motivation to the successful outcome of his rehabilitation programme. There were problems and pitfalls not only for himself in the form of depression, but also for his main carer (his wife, Mandy), who has to cope with personality changes, which are a well-recognised consequence of stroke. Finally, he accurately documents many of the deficiencies in the provision of services for stroke patients in this country, such as inadequate psychological assessment, support and lack of information about stroke for patients and their carers.

Mick Doyle has been an outspoken but constructive critic of Irish rugby and players in recent years. In this book he has been equally honest and critical with himself about his lifestyle, which contributed to this stroke episode. He has taken measures to change his lifestyle, but regrets that he did not do so sooner. He articulates a very clear and important message: stroke is a preventable disease. High blood pressure is the most common treatable risk factor. A combination with smoking or excess alcohol is particularly lethal.

This very personalised narrative, written by an individual who has experienced very contrasting fortunes in life, is a vivid demonstration that stroke may have an excellent outcome. In providing a valuable insight for patients and carers, it will help many to meet the challenges of the most common disabling illness of our time.

Dr Morgan Crowe
(MB, DCH, D. Obst, FRCPI)
Consultant Physician

About the Title

One afternoon Mandy wheeled me out to a quiet spot at the front of Beaumont Hospital. I had come alive about two weeks earlier and was just about able to converse, in a fashion, with my family and friends who came to see me. The sun was warm and the birds were coughing audibly as they sunbathed with apparent abandon, absorbing the sights and sounds all around them; for me, it felt good to just be.

A particular friend, John McInerney, had come to see me, staying for quite a long while; he eventually pushed my wheelchair back to my room. John marvelled at how fortunate I was and how I seemed to have the majority of my faculties still intact. He surprised even me when he said, 'You know, Mick, statistically only about zero point one six per cent of people who suffer a brain haemorrhage, like you, survive; actually the great majority don't get to hospital in time.'

Whatever about the exact accuracy, it is a fact that I have heard of very few people who made it back from my particular problem. However, that explains the title of this book.

The significance of the web and the spider, as background to *Zero Point One Six*, is simply that life may be ambling along, unperturbed and enjoyable, full of action and incident, but

underneath all the gaiety the other life lurks, quiet, ominous and unnoticed, like a spider in its web; it can wait around for ages, and while the web may look artistic, even innocent, as it waits for potential victims, it eventually traps you in its mesh, allowing the tiny weaver to do its damnedest. The finale, when it comes, is sudden and often fatal.

A brain haemorrhage felt just like that to me. It was my web. It scared me to death, almost.

Prologue

A famous songster, and long-time favourite, described so well the whole concept of becoming someone else, with the memorable lines: 'Have you ever heard about the frog who dreamed of being a king/And then became one?'

Although I was obviously in fantasy land when I first became conscious, I was delighted nevertheless to be a king instead of a lowly toad. Still, frog or monarch, it was tempting to keep on inhabiting the land of make-believe that had become spun like a cocoon around me, as I tried to contemplate, most probably like millions of others around the globe, the predicament that had suddenly befallen me. When I was recounting my first fifty years on earth, in the 1991 autobiography *Doyler*, little did I think that I would now be relating this altogether different story. I had felt that my life was charmed, that I was destined to carry on regardless, as usual, almost untouchable. Instead, I was suddenly struck down, almost dead, not so much as a reminder, but more as a short, sharp shock.

I did not have my family properly catered for; I had no legal will drawn up and had little provision made for them for a life without me. In essence, I had made a terrible mess of my life to date really.

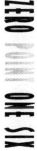

I had suffered a subarachnoid haemorrhage, more simply a brain clot, or a blood clot in that area of the brain where grey matter is said to normally reside.

If you are one of the lucky survivors of a stroke, the immediate overriding feeling is that resembling the futility of a divorce – an overwhelming mood of helplessness and near-failure. Certainly it made me feel as unwanted as a drunk on a motorway, just as unpredictable and as full of danger. This sunburn of inadequacy was soon overtaken by the increasing nagging thoughts of how well I would become if I fought back, what I could expect; would the brain haemorrhage recur and how could I avoid it all happening again and many other niggles as well.

The book speeds through Intensive and Coronary Care, reflects on how I actually got there, lingers a while longer at Rehabilitation and Repair and indulges somewhat more in the recovery of the mind and body at home – and looks with much hope to the future.

Many people have discussed their problems with me; undoubtedly they need to talk to someone who has lived to tell the tale, to articulate their thoughts and fears and the worries that may haunt them, as they did me. And provide some words of help, some practical advice; undoubtedly I felt that there was a huge omission in the whole rehabilitation and recovery process, but that gap between the medical and the laity is now, hopefully, just about narrowing!

Psychology is a funny taskmaster and the deep recesses of the mind literally expand one's mental capabilities, just like a snake's digestive system, to adjust, cope and make progress as it soars to undreamed of heights or plummets to the darkest depths, and, in the process, marginalising all that is peripheral. As with all things in life, the right mental attitude is central – in fact, vital.

My wife Mandy recounts, towards the end of the book, some of her own thoughts and gives her own impressions of the various stages of my illness; a lot of which was new even to me. Her love, and constant presence, like that of son and daughters, Andrew and Emma, Sharon and Amanda, and my dad Michael, who had flown from Morocco, and my brother Tom, was an enormous influence on my steady progress. I owe them and all my family and friends a huge debt. Neither could I ever repay the various surgeons, physicians, nurses, physios and specialists who looked after me. It is all their faults that I am still around . . .

Mick Doyle

ZERO POINT ONE SIX

ONE

As Clear as Mud

I still do not know the exact point at which I first became aware; all I can recall is waking up very gradually and becoming increasingly conscious that I was probably in this world or somewhere else, other than just being dead. I had always envisaged death as blank oblivion; the present overwhelming peace and quiet added considerably to the nothingness. It was all surreal and very frightening. But *where* was I? . . .

My questioning eyes were like a newborn puppy's slowly opening for the first time, as they struggled to focus on the various shapes around me. It felt as if I was in a bright mist which was beginning to lift ever so slightly, where it was difficult to distinguish anything in particular. An overall blur reigned.

In a while I could make out certain fuzzy images – a largish window with daylight streaming through. A room materialised from nowhere, and what looked like at least three or four crazy television sets suddenly appeared, totally unconnected with anything. Still, I could rationalise, when I first became aware of their disjointed presence, that they were attached in some way to the ceiling of the hazy room, set at ridiculous angles from where I was; wherever that was. Shifting my focus nearer home, it quickly became obvious that my eyesight was cockeyed. I seemed

562.196

S0035928

19

to see at least three or four of everything. Shapes were visible, even though I had to guess what some things were. Was I dreaming? Hallucinating?

The next item to attract my sponge-like attention was a symphony of clocks which seemed to hover like Cheshire cats in the air above what must have been some sort of bedside table; the biggest of the clocks made no noise that I could hear, but a hand (it must have been the second hand) measured off time in small silent jumps. Surely, I thought, this must be earth! Is anywhere else like this? Are there clocks in the after-life? Perhaps in purgatory. It looked too normal for hell, though.

In the self-belief that I was still living in this world, my gaze wandered farther afield, as I gained increasingly in confidence, and I could not help noticing that a jumbled matrix of tubes and wires were leading down to me from up there near the ceiling. To me! Blimey, I must have been hooked up to a veritable battery of things, and yet I didn't have a clue where I was or what I was doing there. I was bewildered, but at least alive.

After a while I began to consider my plight and felt reasonably OK; thankfully I didn't experience any pain. I was glad not to be dead, but I was very afraid, of what I didn't exactly know. The unknown loomed like a giant ghost in front of me, in a frightening fog.

As I unconsciously drifted off into a sort of pre-ordained stupor, where life again became suspended, as if the efforts I had made had tired me out, I could hazily remember a sharp pain in my head just before sinking into dark oblivion, in a hospital, seemingly years earlier.

I was alive. But where?

It was later in the day when I next awoke. My eyes were not as blinded by the light, which was still there, but so much less intense now. It was probably summertime, in the late evening. I felt more alive to things around me, more in touch, not as disorientated as the last time. I now had a previous time to relate to, a definite focal point, and suddenly I was feeling more secure about myself. I was still fairly hazy about where I was, but it must have been in a room in some house, safe out of the shadows, those fathomless ghouls that I could sense lurking outside the window.

A feeling of numbness prevailed, though there were no real pains. While more objects around me took on much greater clarity and meaning, I was still, subconsciously, imprisoned inside a sort of bubble which was definitely not unpleasant; but overwhelming emotions of blankness surrounded and consumed me. It felt as if I was a compliant guest somewhere; that was it – a guest, a patient. Patient! That meant that I must have been sick at some stage; nurses must have cared for me and doctors must have toiled over me with their almost studied nonchalance. It didn't bear thinking about. Was I a helpless vegetable?

I was now, though, well and truly their prisoner – unable to do very much. Whatever acted as a prompt, perhaps it was fear, made me move my head around, and I tried to zoom in on something. I could rationalise at least that I was in a bed, that the floor looked miles away and that the walls and doors more or less melted indiscriminately into each other. A chair or two stood in silent vigil against the walls; these kept moving in and out ever so slightly and apart from the by-now familiar television sets and the scrambled mass of tubes going to and coming from somewhere, very little else registered.

I was wearing a kind of plain white smock and could feel that my unshaven facial hair had grown into the makings of a beard; I must have been unconscious for a few weeks to sprout such a burgeoning fungus.

But why was my eyesight so poor? It had never been like that before. I knew that I wore glasses for extreme light and distances, but previously I used to see very well without them. What had happened to me? Was it connected in some way with the pain that I had remembered the last time I was awake? Where was Mandy? Where was everybody? Why was it so quiet? Eerie, like a graveyard.

Thank God at least that I was alone. I didn't really want to meet anybody but Mandy just yet. There was no sound at all except for the barely perceptible movement of the second hands of the clocks and some distant muffling. The clocks – they were still there – all eleven of them. They were haunting me like those ghost-like television sets, following me around. I was perplexed and confused.

Suddenly it hit me like the sudden shock of lightning, or else I was dreaming: I was hooked up to such an array of tubes and wires, seemingly running in all directions, that I resembled a set of bagpipes, even to my distorted vision. I must have looked like an alien being who had been dredged up from the innermost fjords of Steven Spielberg's imagination.

There was a tube from my nose leading to some kind of plastic bag, which in turn appeared to be hanging from a stand beside my bed. That must have been a stomach tube or an intravenous drip. If I had been unconscious for any length of time, then I couldn't feed myself, could I? That was that problem sorted out. I had heard all about stomach tubes before, but this was personal experience, no mere correspondence course.

Moving downwards gingerly, almost fearfully, I felt around and found some wires leading to my chest; these must have been monitors of some sort, to keep track of my various functions. My fingertips by this stage were on fire, hypersensitive and impatiently waiting to explore further along my person. The indignity of it all! But worse was to follow; apart from a few tubes leading from my arms to another stand, I felt a plastic tube going into my willie – it had to have been a urethral tube – obviously to cater for weeing while I slept. Was I incontinent?

There were a few other probes wired up to my chest, ankles and arms to complete my humiliation. I was a patient all right. All that, plus the fact that the bedclothes were wrapped fairly tightly about me, ensured that I could not move around very much, as if a restraining straitjacket was keeping me immobile like a newborn baby in its cot. Why did cot deaths keep suggesting themselves to me? I felt that if all the intimate details about me had been recorded somewhere, then I would have hated to be the one to interpret them. Anyway, I was glad I didn't have to.

The haze in the room gradually lifted, becoming a bit clearer with time; though the now fewer television sets and clocks were still placed at daft angles. The walls were cream-coloured, the doors, ceiling and window were white, and the floor was covered in linoleum. The chairs were lying up against the walls as before, like mute sentries, and a solitary light bulb shone down from the ceiling.

Near the bed were a cupboard with a few cards on the top, a shelf full of nothing and a closet. The stand and the plastic bags on hooks were floating somewhere over the cupboard. I didn't hear anybody come in or go out of the room – they must have thought that I was still in the Land of Nod, sound asleep and counting sheep.

A whole jumble of questions formed a queue, jostling to be posed, and I actually looked forward to meeting somebody, sometime. Could I talk to them? I didn't know. I tried to practise by conversing with myself, like a half-idiot, but no sound came out. I was like a mime artist fluent in Braille.

Sleep inexorably overcame me.

I once knew a second-hand car salesman (I presume he sold cars first-hand, too) who was always full of devilment; his eyes would twinkle with merriment whenever he described some major feature about the car he was currently flogging. He never bent the truth much, mind you, but nevertheless he put his own inimitable spin on it.

'This car doesn't actually start in the morning,' he would say, 'it just commences.' At least nobody could ever accuse Vincent Keane of deceit. It was when he got bolder, continuing his monologue, that one became baffled at the direction his prattle was taking. 'The back seat was rarely used,' he said, 'and the car was never driven at night.' Usually by then anyone not interested in buying a car from him would have found something else to do.

When I eventually regained consciousness after four weeks of comatose suspension of living, I was only just about able to 'commence' as well. I made haste very slowly, contenting myself with becoming *au fait* with my immediate surroundings.

I am now aware, of course, that there were many times when I acted as if I was conscious (but wasn't) and sometimes exhibited bizarre behaviour during my first four weeks of postponed animation in Intensive Care. I honestly don't recall any of that; whatever I did during this period were not conscious acts on my part, and while I don't actually blame myself, I cannot pin these incidents on someone else either. However, my family never lets me forget them.

Sometime in those early days of being awake, things became significantly different. It was like Disneyland on Viagra – everything was huge; Mickey Mouse was enormous, Donald Duck was like an ostrich, Tom and Jerry took on the shapes of an elephant and a lion, while poor old Flipper looked like a large whale! Even the angels, fairies and elves were out of this world, as they looked down on me while I fiddled around on my own, getting accustomed to my surroundings. They were always there, even if I tried to blink, with their silhouettes moving in and out of the shadows, receding from view as they merged into nothingness.

I didn't realise at that stage exactly how much the medical staff had had to do just to keep me alive. Obviously when you wake up after being 'dead' for a long while, you do not really appreciate how much has been done for you while you were asleep. It was hugely exciting to be alive, and I was filled with an overwhelming sense of relief and gratitude for the chance even to see things again.

Pretty soon I took the opportunity to become composed, marshal my thoughts and self-motivate, as I steeled myself to meet other people whom I could not avoid: obviously these would be a lot of strange nurses and doctors, in addition, of course, to my family and friends. I laughed inwardly and almost, but not quite, mentally apologised to many people for denying them a good funeral and many booze-ups during the whole ritual of death. Possibly some folks were even disappointed! They will now have to wait for a while longer.

Soon a tea lady with a trolley materialised, saying something incoherent. Didn't she know about me? Apparently not. She was probably asking me if I wanted anything; when I didn't appear to answer (how could I with a tube stuck in my face?), she shuffled off leaving tea and a biscuit behind her.

It was morning when she removed the stale meal. (This whole episode was replayed monotonously – meals being left unattended, unasked for and generally with the frustrated, hungry patient being unaware of their presence. It was amazing but continued for the time I was in Beaumont.)

The fatigued breakfast told me that it was mid-morning; otherwise I wouldn't have had a clue. It was an expensive way of telling the time. However, I still didn't know exactly what had happened or how I had come to be there. I would find out soon enough.

ZERO POINT ONE SIX

TWO

A Bolt from the Grey

A well-known song had often cautioned, 'That's life, that's what all the people say, flyin' high in April, shot down in May'; except in my case, it had been delayed until Sunday, 14 July 1996 – and then it came as some surprise. But why me?

I knew, of course, that during the previous twelve months I had squeezed a fair wedge of action into a hectic life. I had more Sky Miles than anyone in *Star Trek*. For example, in June 1995 I had served as a member of Irish Television's sports panel, covering the third Rugby World Cup in South Africa (which the new South Africa won, to the huge delight of many people).

The nation was led by the ebullient Nelson Mandela. The President was an incredible sight, dressed in a South African rugby jersey, particularly since he was being beamed on television around the world. It was uplifting to see his unrestrained vigour and joy, his blackness fitting in so perfectly with the comparative whiteness of the South African captain François Pinnaer. The major significance of the Springboks' Rugby World Cup success was that it signalled to the world that the hateful regime of apartheid was finally at an end.

I had also flown to Atlanta, Omaha, São Paulo, Mexico and New Zealand during the year to help launch our company's dairy

ZERO POINT ONE SIX

hygiene product, Agrisept, finally holidaying with Mandy and daughter Emma in the major Grand Cayman Island, in June 1996, for about three weeks. Grand Cayman Rugby Club had invited me to speak at their annual dinner and to enjoy the sights for a while. Our holiday there with Alan and Gloria Russell, now married and living in Limerick, was unforgettable.

I had already spent days on end in London stimulating corporate interest in our developing company; it was all worthwhile.

And so with all the toing and froing, I had barely had time to draw breath, relax, take stock and plan the company's future once we had welcomed the new shareholders on board, when life decided that it was time to end all this madness; I was to be taught not only a hard lesson but one hell of a timely one, too.

The late, great John Lennon once remarked, in one of his more lucid moments, 'Life's what happens to you when you're makin' plans.' That's exactly what happened to me. Me! How dare it?

The day before it happened, 13 July, began as a lovely, pleasant summer day; we had been wired up for Sky TV on the previous day and I wanted to watch Saturday's live rugby test between Australia and South Africa at eleven o'clock. Since the card to operate the system was still log-jammed in the postal service, I watched the game on TV at Mulvey's Emporium, in Naas, my local watering-hole, drinking a bottle of fine French red and a few pints of beer afterwards with some mates – just to wash down the wine and round off the morning, so to speak.

Afterwards I enjoyed a barbecue with Mandy, Andrew and Emma during that afternoon; I drank even more wine (I must have thought that I was a guest at the marriage feast of Caana). Later on that evening I listened to Eric Clapton, Pete Townshend and Roger Daltrey on the television – they were brilliant, vivid reminders of an era long gone.

For me, there still remains a big gap in memory between the barbecue and the rock stars. Perhaps it was a portent. Anyway, I went to bed happily, taking a few aspirins for a drink-induced headache, to make sure that it would be gone by morning – as it usually was.

I slept the sleep of peace, without a care in the world, looking forward to Sunday, hoping for a fine day and dreaming perhaps of all the usual leisurely pursuits of suntan-lotion weather. But instead of the summer morning delights I had anticipated, I ended up with the identical headache to the night before, knowing instinctively, like pet dogs can sense your imminent departure on holiday, that I was in serious trouble. The pain in my head, which should have been past tense by now, was something else altogether. I cannot remember having any other warning signs, or ones that I heeded anyway.

Looking back now, from the high moral perch of the know all, I am amazed at how naïve I had been, how ridiculously stupi l. I must have really thought to myself, I'm invincible; nothing bad will ever happen to me. But the pain had, by degrees, progressed from bad to terrible. It became far more insistent, and therefore worrying, as it travelled along its pre-ordained route, like a creeping, menacing reptile, progressing from a dull ache, past the signpost signalling a more pronounced but somehow more diffuse, less focused thumper, finally to where the screaming agony of my head being on fire revealed all the naked grating of hypersensitive nerve endings.

I could hardly stand it, never having had a pain even approaching this level of intensity. It felt as if an ever-tightening band had settled around my forehead, which was dripping wet. My mouth was watering copiously, too. I must have been suffering a combination of rapidly escalating fear and the helplessness of almost total resignation, jumbled up like a breakfast bowl of home-made muesli, together with this head-splitting pain; I was also hyperventilating uncontrollably.

I pulled on a much-worn tracksuit, and wandered out on to

the back lawn, for what I did not really know; I was probably trying to avoid the unravelling reality of what was happening to me: to escape. Pretty soon I was drenched in a perspiration that seemed to be limitless, like being caught unawares with a window open in a car wash. My facial muscles began to experience a weird sensation which I couldn't control: a sort of numbness, like paraesthesia, following a visit to the dentist – except that this kind of dental numbness wears off quickly.

My eyesight had deteriorated rapidly to where it had obviously gone off on tour, leaving me feeling frightened and vulnerable. My spectacles on the lounge table (where I had left them the night before) wouldn't have been of any use in this situation. I knew where familiar objects should be, just about, and grabbed the chain-link fence surrounding the lawn, to keep my balance, as I poked around somewhat like an aged lover going about his business by touch, or by memory. Soon I felt very wobbly, stumbling around like a blind man, wandering about trying to find his bearings. What the hell was happening to me?

Mandy and Emma, naturally, were afraid and confused, realising that I was in trouble, and not knowing what to do; the poor old dogs couldn't understand what was going on either. Both their worries for me and fears of an unknown future, which must have passed across their vision like fast-forwarding video adverts, were mirrored by abject terror on my part and the disbelieving fright at the vista that was unfolding.

Shortly after that, I recall lying flat on the now reclining front seat of our car, with Emma sitting behind Mandy as she drove. We were on our way to our medical locum's house as our own GP was away for the weekend. What an inappropriate time for me to fall ill, I thought foolishly, or for him to be missing.

By this stage my head had almost unbelievably become even more painful, accompanied by increasing tension, unlike anything I had previously experienced. I began moaning, I remember, and couldn't get out of the car at the doctor's surgery, but realised that I knew John Keagh very well; this made me feel even more of a fool. Straightaway, he suggested that we go to the Casualty Department of the local hospital in Naas. I must have looked terrible, nearly dead by then.

Somehow, how I don't know, I ended up on a bed in the Casualty Department, with anxious faces peering at me. I faintly remember telling some medic with a stethoscope, bending over me, as he tried to figure out what my symptoms actually meant, that 'My heart is fine, thanks; it's my bloody head that hurts me, but for God's sake don't go near it.' Fear and frustration were the two cardinal signs by this time.

Everything after that was and is a complete blank. My family filled in the pieces for me long afterwards. I'm glad I missed it all, but they couldn't and didn't; they saw it all in vivid technicolour.

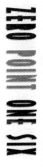
ZERO POINT ONE SIX

THREE

A New Awakening

Standing alone on the shores of a giant pothole, I was safe for the moment but fearful of venturing further into inhospitable territory. Apart from my funny eyesight, things were becoming clearer by the minute, as if a mist was gradually lifting, propelling me into contact with what was going on around me, and making me more aware of the hidden dangers of the pothole and its satellites.

A pleasant voice from near the door asked if I would be taking 'breakfast this morning – tea, toast? What about porridge?' Was the meals' lady speaking to *me*? Quickly realising that there was nobody else in the room, I nodded a 'Yes, please.'

Pulling the special feeding trolley up over me in the bed, she deposited her load cheerily and left, pushing her food cart along with a song on her lips. She obviously needed a bright outlook and positive attitude to keep up her spirits.

Then it suddenly struck me: I couldn't manage to eat or drink by myself. I was still hooked up to all those tubes and bags, being fed by stomach tube, and the odd drip. Surely she must have seen, but obviously did not. Looking wildly around, I noticed the fully opened curtains and the clouds scudding across a blue sky. The weather looked warm. How could I tell? I didn't really know

ZERO POINT ONE SIX

for sure, but it didn't feel cold with my window partly open; the room wasn't arctic and neither was I. Then it dawned on me that someone had been in my room earlier while I was asleep and had noiselessly drawn the curtains to a new day. I was glad they had; the *new-day* symbolism wasn't lost on me either – I was already beginning to feel like a new person; it was contagious, like a head cold. The brain was still working.

Looking wistfully down at the food before me, I resigned myself to not eating for a while longer, located a buzzer and pressed the button. A nurse came almost straightaway, took in the incongruous scene and burst out laughing. I couldn't blame her, but regretfully I wasn't able to let the same raucous explosion of release out of me, together with all the pent-up frustration that I felt; I had to be content instead with a mere gurgle, so as not to dislodge anything. Even a simple laugh was a potential catastrophe. What a way to be!

The nurse left, laughing, saying that she'd be back with a gang. That sounded ominously like a crowd of muggers, but I needn't have worried. A doctor and two other nurses returned with her soon after and in no time at all the tubes and wires lay redundant – my body was a temple once more, inviolate, and it was also operating under its own power.

All the tubes and wires were suddenly discarded like worn-out needles, having long since done their jobs expertly while I was out cold. I wasn't sorry to see the back of them, though. At least that was the first pothole negotiated safely. One down and many more to go. The only road for me to take was forward and up, for now.

The breakfast was stone cold by this stage, the porridge looking like set concrete. Someone brought me a plate of hot toast and fresh tea instead.

Afterwards, as I lay back to rest, I noticed that the TV was turned on to a sports channel. At breakfast time? I turned up the sound via the remote control on the locker top and found that the programme was all about the Olympic Games in Atlanta, Georgia. (I had been a visitor there, in a previous life, and had loved the place. I had a great flush of nostalgia about all the trips I had made there, to the South-Eastern Conventions in the Omni building, then owned by Aer Lingus).

It must have been pre-recorded – who would be running around like maniacs this early? However, I couldn't see the pictures properly, even with my eyes scrunched up squinting; but I recognised many familiar names, felt quite at home and lowered the sound to just barely audible.

With the recognisable and welcome voices on the television and the steady crack of the starting pistol, together with the regular blast of anthems, acting as a soothing background, I slipped into an easy sleep, dreaming of Mandy. She would probably come to see me today. I hadn't laid seeing-eyes on her for such a long time; certainly not without all these tubes sticking out of me at odd angles. I must have looked like a demented octopus to her.

I woke up, desperate to go to the toilet; I pressed the buzzer again, but now with far more urgency. I almost began to wish that the urethral tube was still in place and that I could have piddled in my sleep; but I quickly banished that unworthy thought. Things weren't that bad yet. Shane, my nurse and main helper, came in answer to my blast on the bell and very patiently helped a very unsteady 'resident' to the bathroom.

He was a godsend; we both tried valiantly to make me presentable for Mandy's expected visit. As you can imagine, Shane did most of the work. I was incredibly wobbly and couldn't stand or walk unaided.

Looking into the bathroom mirror for the first time since I

had come there, I was taken aback; a crazy wild-eyed stranger was staring back at me. I had changed. It was quite a shock – there's no delicate way to put it. Blunt is probably best. I quickly turned away, and was led back to the bed.

Despite all Shane's patient help and encouragement, the exertions in the toilet had left me drained, but I had proved at least that I could make it to the bathroom, and even though my eyesight was severely hampered I could talk in a sort of fashion. I had crossed the Rubicon of yet another pothole without mishap. Would Mandy recognise me?

Luckily, my concerns about our first meeting were clearly misplaced; its newness was like our first date all over again. Thank God for that. We were both quite shy initially, reserved even.

My trip to hospital had obviously changed many things irrevocably. It felt great just to be alive, even if I was lying helpless in this bed, with my wife bending over me, holding me tight, murmuring quietly and soothing my face. How I longed to be the one doing the holding; I wanted to wrap her in the warm embrace of my aching arms and squeeze tight.

Both of us were thrilled to meet again and couldn't stop kissing. We sought the release of crying, and were quickly joined by a very shy Emma, instantly becoming a threesome once more. We must have presented a weird tableau of tears and talk, wonderment and kisses; a family again and I truly loved them. Everything felt great once more, definitely worth being alive for.

The process of getting to know each other, all over again, was really beginning in earnest, even though much remained unsaid for the moment. Many stored-up questions, about Andrew, Sharon and Amanda, our parents, the business, the *Sunday Independent*, for which I used to write, friends and events and the like, were discussed somehow, but our minds were preoccupied with ourselves. We looked at each other – like we were unreal, searching each other's faces for any signs of negatives.

Mandy and Emma looked great to me. I was almost speechless seeing them and more than just glad that I had made it back from the near-eternity of death. Their love was a powerful motivation.

They left after that first short visit, promising to return again the next day – like they did every day after that. I felt like a cat with a saucer of milk, except it was more like a bucket of the stuff. I had been afraid quite a long time ago, before I passed out, that I might never see them on earth again; but now I could, thank the Lord.

With happy thoughts and a barrow full of plans for the future, I drifted off into a dreamland that had no sheep, no ghosts in it, but lots of sea, swimming pools, cars and food. It suddenly reminded me of Lanzarote, where Mandy, Emma and I had spent such memorable holidays. It was great to be a complete person again, at the start of a new life. But I was, and I had; wasn't I the lucky one?

Counting sheep was only for insomniacs – or shepherds.

As I lay back in bed, twiddling my thumbs, my thoughts left me and took off skywards on magic carpets of their own. My mind, their parent, became their fellow-traveller, wafting along with them in the ether. Something kept prompting me to unravel their hidden meaning, pregnant with explanation, about to give birth.

Thanking my lucky stars that I would now be looking down at the daisies rather than up, I began to change my vision to a sharper focus and, as I concentrated, I began to rationalise how I actually ended up there, in this mess. How had I descended so low; what had happened? My thoughts, at last, were becoming free of all constraints; they *would* be untangled this time.

I knew by now, of course, that the final precipitating push over the gaping edge was a brain haemorrhage – a bleeding of the subarachnoid part of the brain, which more or less proved that the body had absorbed so much punishment and shock that it had come to the end of its tether. And yet, I felt uneasily, guiltily, that there was still more baggage hidden away somewhere in the dark recesses, and that something else kept impelling me to face up to the true facts and admit the primary predisposing cause of my descent. There was to be no bluffing this time, no hiding.

As if to postpone the inevitable, my fertile mind was wildly searching around for excuses, trying desperately to sidestep the real cause, instead of staring it down; but the stark reality of the hospital in which I was now a resident focused my thinking processes, like a guillotine concentrates the mind, denying me the luxury of trying to convert futile apologias into valid reasons – instead, forcing me to accept the truth.

Truth was obviously to be the new game from now on, with no escape. The straitjacket of conscience had made me confront the unpalatable at long last; I couldn't escape to somewhere else: I was in Beaumont Hospital, by extremely lucky circumstance, because I had lived for too long in the outside lane of life's motorway, 'doin' the ton', my right foot flooring the accelerator. That's why!

It was as direct and as simple as that. All that waffle about 'pressures of work' and the intelligent-sounding mumbo-jumbo of 'occupational hazards' wouldn't wash this time, because I knew only too well what had driven me to this state: me, a patient all of a sudden, and the new me was not in joking mode any longer.

The brain haemorrhage had made me far more direct. It had galvanised me, and whatever about my other faculties, my mind was crystal clear. It was like the clarity I had often experienced, in the past, in that period just before alcohol dulled the senses.

Being brutally candid with myself, in this new mood of openness, taking an almost masochistic delight in frankness without frivolities, I mentally admitted to being excessively overweight, overstressed and overindulgent of the booze. I had been shoving the bâteau out for too long, too far from the safety of the shore, and not only was I intent on melting the candle at either end, I felt compelled to set fire to the middle as well. The midnight oil had long since been used up; even the warning light had fused and gone out. I was in one hell of a mess.

The alarm gong had been sounded in 1987, when I had experienced a heart-attack in Auckland, New Zealand, during the first Rugby World Cup competition. Almost unbelievably I had ignored it, heeding its message for only a few months, until the fear itself had left me and the sudden fright of the coronary incident had rapidly become a distant memory. An uncomfortable reminder, it was locked away in a conveniently forgotten pigeon hole.

Unfortunately for me, I did not take stock at the time and slow down, giving myself even a sporting chance, just as the friendly Auckland cardiologist had advised me. I deluded myself that I knew better, relapsing instead, almost with alacrity, into a never-ending spiral of self-gratification, absorbing all the action around me like a paper towel.

Oblivious to the real truth, I was also fooling myself into believing that I was really living well, enjoying a good quality of life. What, me, an alcoholic? No way! Sure, I did *like* a drink and would readily concede that I was a heavy drinker. But an alcoholic; the thought always horrified me.

But the inexorably tightening tentacles of the liquid demon lulled me, an otherwise intelligent human being, into thinking that I could handle most situations easily, giving up the booze whenever I needed to. Take it, or leave it. Easy. After all, wasn't I incredibly strong willed? I was, like hell. Not where drink was concerned.

The grip of the innocent-looking, socially acceptable booze proved it was a formidable adversary; often a companion but always my controller! I hadn't started to drink seriously until after the summer of 1968, towards the end of my international rugby career, playing on the British Lions Rugby Union Tour to South Africa. I was then twenty-eight.

Even though some joker had put vodka into my Coke during birthday celebrations in Cape Town, I had never been tempted to drink during my rugby years; I very definitely made up for lost time since. I took to it like a mouse to cheese, after first becoming accustomed to the huge change from Coke to beer. I had come a long way since the night I drank eighteen pints of Coca-Cola when I qualified as a vet. What a sea-change!

After a hesitant start, under the expert tutelage of the late Pat Taffe, the famous Arkle's legendary mentor, taking a drink soon became a way of life for me; it felt natural. Far from interfering with my lifestyle, drinking became a natural part of it, proving so easy to succumb to and almost impossible to avoid. I was reluctant to dispense with the supporting cast of the bottle and the glass. Why should I? To be perfectly honest, I liked it just fine.

First in rugby and latterly in everyday circles, the culture of booze was traditional, normally expected and almost unavoidable. It was always pleasant, enjoyable. While it wasn't declared a drink-free occasion, the pre-match period was one of relative constraint and common sense – total abstinence on the day leading up to every game was the usual routine, for the players and myself as coach, at any rate.

However, when all the pressure was off, the game finished and everything tidied up and dusted, we generally let our hair down (those of us who still had hair) and gave the gargle a fair old lash. The Leinster team won quite a lot of matches then, to add that extra fillip to our celebrations, giving us a valid reason to go wild. Losing a match still provided an excuse to consume drink, but it was nothing like the buzz that winning generated, no matter how you drowned your disappointments.

Whenever the team wins, everybody is in good humour, endlessly drinking and socialising; but losing is demeaning and often humiliating. Unfortunately, from the carousing point of view, I saw very little of this side. The culture of the scapegoat is alive and swimming near the surface when you have been vanquished, and drink, even to excess, to camouflage your sorrows, is only a temporary overcoat, a poor one at that.

It often occurred to me that I drank too much in between the regular weekends on the rugby calendar, constantly looking forward to meeting all my mates and fellow-travellers again, regularly. Rugby occasions certainly did lend themselves to drinking, being tailor-made for carousing far away from spouses, and behaviour often became riotous on after-match occasions; it was never destructive or nasty, mind you. There was never anything to regret.

I was married to Lynne during this time; while a rugby fan, she accepted my love-affair with rugby without ever becoming deeply involved. Being a Bristol rugby club lady member meant that she knew all about the drinking marathons that often ensued after serious rugby weekends and so, apart from coming along with me on the odd occasion, she generally stayed away.

The whole representative rugby roadshow attracted me tremendously: the jokes, the anecdotes and all the ridiculous unadult-type behaviour, which outsiders would probably consider infantile. In fact the conviviality of male company, and that of the wives and girlfriends, after matches, and of bridging that gap between the current youth and our own earlier generation drew me like a moth to light.

Once again, I was able to re-live my own rugby career through all the modern great players, ensuring this time around that they would be freed by me, their coach, of all the shackles of conservatism, able to express fully their God-given talents, which as players we were not encouraged to do; this was a different era.

For three years around 1990 I had temporarily quit, drinking

low-alcohol beer instead. I did this of my own volition, as well as heeding the prompts of a few friends. Emma was due to make her world entry in July 1989, and Mandy and I were to be married in Omagh in March of that year. I wanted to be in great shape for both of them. That at least was the plan. It had been quite a struggle, but certainly worth it; I felt much better. Still, I knew that I would begin again some day.

Pretty soon, the previous hedonistic lifestyle of booze and self-indulgence beckoned, like a seductive temptress. Of course my attempts at moderation never really had a chance of permanency. I hadn't changed my social pattern at all. I was still frequenting old familiar watering-holes and associating with the same drinking mates as before – I really didn't want to be without their company; after all, the camaraderie and the buzz were the reasons why I was such a social drinker in the first place. It was a serious compulsion.

Falling into similar, well-worn routines again, like favourite slippers, I consumed drink with abandon and even new-found fervour (making up for three 'lost' years?). Drink revealed only its friendly nature, never threatening me; I had become the respectable face of booze. Gargle had become the gasoline that fuelled my engine.

The ease with which I could take in copious amounts of drink, and the stealthy manner in which it had surreptitiously permeated my whole life, surprised even me; it certainly frightened me. Lunch-time meals often became occasions for a few gins, a few more whiskies and the odd bottle of wine; just enough not to fall asleep during the afternoon. After daily work finished, a time regularly welcomed by at least two hours of wine and Guinness, Jameson whiskey and chat, all the usual examples of companionship and bonhomie received their due 'physical-fitness' regimens.

In fact life seemed to settle down to a full timetable of work and socialising, though my work could never be misconstrued as mundane; I was Chairman and Managing Director of Biojen

International plc, basically a company selling products for animal health. This entailed extensive involvement in scientific correspondence, marketing and technical support and endless days and thousands of miles of travel; cities and time zones became just items on a long itinerary. In spite of all this, it was tremendously enjoyable and satisfying.

My office was in Naas, about three miles from home. I lived with Mandy and Emma in a charming old stone cottage out in the countryside in Sherlockstown, near Sallins in County Kildare, with a beautiful view across the wide fields of the Wicklow hills. Horses, cattle and sheep graze the lush grass. The scene is all so rustic, idyllic really.

I had a good home life, but I know now, because Mandy has told me, whenever I press her, that I missed out on so much of it by not being there. Of course I was off enjoying the company of my drinking friends instead of that of my wife and new baby. I utterly regret that now but I'm truly grateful that I *only* ever stayed away, needlessly; thank God I never became abusive on booze. I would never be able to face myself clearly if I had descended to that low level.

And so, while my everyday experiences were always varied, life did assume a sort of humdrum aspect. I suppose it was relieved by writing my weekly article on rugby, mostly for the *Sunday Independent*. I had gone to watch games all over Ireland, Britain and France, meeting many friends and acquaintances. I'd had a memorable time; of course the delights of drinking were savoured to the full on these 'historic' occasions. In reality life seemed to settle around work, travel, family life and sports – with drink everywhere. While I felt that I could juggle all my lives, I know deep down that my capacity for socialising, and the countless opportunities everyday living presented of it, really worried me, prodding my senses of saner times.

Often the nagging suggestion that I should take it easy clamoured for attention in my conscious mind, but in vain. In many a sane moment, not just waking up full of remorse and the usual morning-after-the-night-before resolutions, I realised that my life was slowly, but definitely, slipping away from me.

My friend Dr Morgan Crowe had been so right, so often. What a pity I didn't heed his advice. I heard him, believed him and understood him, but the selfishness of alcohol made me ignore his sound warnings. Life really became a liar, promising so much, delivering so little. I just didn't seem able to do anything about the direction in which I was headed. I don't believe I wanted to either. You can lead a horse to water, but . . .

The drink, though hugely enjoyable, was quietly ambushing my days, forming too large a part in the overall relaxation process. It was frightening how quickly the weeks merged into each other and flew by, as if they had never happened. I certainly noticed all that, but did nothing about it. It was critically important that I should change my tune, but unfortunately I didn't. The addiction owned my resolve too; I just let everything drift, observing but not bothering.

Work, as far as I could rationalise, hadn't suffered up to 1996, but life and love were definitely passing me by, with increasing rapidity, either with only a sideswipe at my conscience or else a cursory nod. It was all so fleeting, like the life-cycle of a butterfly.

Unfortunately, drink made me incredibly self-centred, subconsciously to disregard anything that might be even slightly related to the future, like behaving responsibly towards one's developing family, and concentrate instead on the enjoyment of the here and now. Even though it was the last thing on my mind, or ever in my intentions, I sidelined my young wife and daughter, pushing them to the edges of my drinking life as I 'allowed' them to assume secondary roles, while they were left to fend for themselves. It wasn't a sin of commission, but it definitely was one of omission. What a stupid, blind fool I was! Self-gratification had made me numb to reality.

I was missing out on so many things at home and, worst of all,

I was oblivious to it. I revelled in the role of the macho male, passively allowing the bonhomie in my life to cloud my true perspective of normality: like socialising less, drinking far less and spending more time at home. Drink had become my constant companion, my friend. Where would I be without it; or what would I be instead of it? It had completely taken over my very existence.

Fortunately, at long last, I have now jettisoned all that unwanted luggage that had been weighing me down for so long, finally admitting, in fact readily accepting, that I *did* have a serious problem. It was some intoxicating drink disorder!

I had quit smoking previously on National No Smoking Day in 1982, cigarettes, pipes, cigars, dried tea – the lot; I had unsuccessfully tried many times before, with the usual result, soon back heavier on the smokes than ever.

On this particular occasion, though, I had carefully prepared myself, counting down the days, marking them off until the specific get-off-the-pot day. I actually relished the ending of a long affair with tobacco, preparing to become eventually free of its poisons and fatal attractions. I have no doubt now that a positive mental attitude conquered my fuming habits, helping me to overcome the withdrawal symptoms I had obviously suffered, keeping my determination focused firmly on the main objective. On this occasion I *had* meant business. Two major events helped my final decision: my young daughter, Sharon, asked me to give up fags, and the wheezing from emphysema did not appeal to me.

It wasn't all pain though. I became aware of a few new advantages: interestingly enough, I found out that I had far fewer surges of the usual adrenalin during provincial rugby games (I was coaching Leinster at the time); I suffered from fewer stress-induced headaches, during and after these games, and, wonder of

ZERO POINT ONE SIX

wonders, I could drink more, for longer, without becoming inebriated.

Sugar had probably been among my first obsessions to bite the dust. I loved the stuff. I took it in almost everything.

I had started using sugar-like tablets as substitutes in my tea and coffee at first (not that I needed them but because it was fashionable), but then I packed the whole lot in. Perhaps they helped me initially to conquer the craving; I don't know but I'll give them the benefit of the doubt. But the sugar that is inherent in most foods is far more insidious, lying in wait for the innocent; as I found out much later.

The gargle therefore wasn't the only potential banana skin in my life. I almost wish it had been; it may have been easier to overcome just the one addiction. But stress and the overconsumption of good food represented serious obstacles along the path of life. I didn't stuff myself, mark you, on ready-food or convenience quickies. I never became partial to munching on the move or aspired to becoming a burger king.

I just ate far too much of even the 'correct' food and, in paying simultaneous lip-service to avoiding occasions of real stress, I blindly embraced the hectic lifestyle, with welcoming arms akimbo. Gradually I became as unfit as a beached whale; my GP's alarm, frowns and his regular chats with me made eminent sense, but only at the time, temporarily filling me with the resolve to change my ways.

All the prodding or even subtle suggestions that I take myself to task turned out like all good intentions – I talked a good game, but did not play one. I was an expert, a non-playing captain! High blood pressure and high cholesterol levels did not seem to register with me; they made little difference. Finally, they almost claimed me.

Wasn't excess in all things part and parcel of a competitive, type-A personality anyway, and moderation something that one bought in a sex shop? Looking back at it all now, with the clarity of hindsight, I realised full well, as sure as I was confined to this hospital bed, having suffered a brain haemorrhage, that the madcap life had to stop. Either I packed in the drink, not just cut it down, while drastically reducing all the other excesses at the same time, or I would end up dead. That was the unpalatable but inescapable choice.

A life in which booze and food featured so negatively wasn't really a terribly exciting proposition, but it was looming ever so large on the screen of my life. I realised that I couldn't support the whole hectic routine; the 'now and again' had become 'again and again'. My drinking had progressed from the occasional to the regular. It had ceased being fun; it was enjoyable, but not fun any more.

Something obviously had to give, and it was me. It had taken a dangerous brain haemorrhage to bring me to the edge of sanity, as I considered all the dangers of a suddenly uncertain future. Escapism was now a dirty word after what I had gone through, and I could never again contemplate a return to my former lifestyle.

FOUR

Many Shadows

My guardian angel, an experienced hand by now (who probably often wished to be off guarding someone else, somebody more predictable), was not alone faced with a new kind of dilemma, but he also had to act for me, as if by proxy, during my prolonged 'sleep' and for the first months of mental struggles. My body during this time was trying to repair itself; it must have considered each day at a time to be a major achievement. The will to live is truly incredible. Meanwhile, my mind cavorted with fairies; innocently, I hope.

I have always envisaged this unseen figure to be a 'he'; surely a 'she' would blush to the very roots of her hair if she found herself in a men's toilet, or in a male changing room – or whatever! Could she survive a ruck, where macho males regularly act out their caveman heritage, or an equally male hormone-dominated brawl in football? She probably would have long since buzzed off to become a security guard somewhere less explosive. And so I presumed it was, and is, a he and that we were of a similar age. How has he since aged, I often wondered?

Enough of this drivel. At any rate, my guardian angel was left to his own devices for a few precarious months, acting out Mandy's and all the rest of my family's wishes too, keeping me

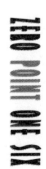

safe and alive. But as soon as I could rationalise a bit for myself, my guardian angel, like a good Man Friday, melted back into the woodwork and, apart from the odd word of encouragement, stayed quiet.

However, my shadow, my alter ego, took over my life and dominated it whenever it could. It moved ahead of me, like with an early motoring vehicle, acting like a filter for those first few months when I had difficulty clinging on to this world. It was much larger than me then and for the most part prompted me to think survival rather than repair and recovery. I couldn't do much else anyway in those early days.

Basically, the overwhelming feelings back then were *thankfulness* for the second chance; sorrow for the things I had lost, seemingly irretrievably; an overwhelming desire to hang on to life and a determination to adjust, in whatever way was best, and hopefully *improve*.

My wife and I thought as one and, even though I may have been a thundering nuisance and as awkward as a bag of fighting cats, she either removed or kept hidden all the external hassles from me, allowing me to concentrate on the job in hand. She would intelligently keep all outside pressures away from me. I was lucky; I owe her.

Naturally I was totally introverted then, zeroing in on everything around me in hospital and paying little real attention to much else. My concentration span was limited and I don't recall many faces or events from those early weeks.

I often had weird nightmares, or else disconcerting dreams: like of one visitor seducing all round him (adding to his 'accomplishments') while the female spouse of another tried to influence the nursing staff, to wheedle secrets about my actual state out of them. I have mentally apologised to both of them, and they'll never know either how lucky they were to escape uncensored.

Many things had become routine, like temperature and blood pressure readings, trips to the toilet, washing myself in the bathroom and so forth. I had let my beard grow for only the second time in my life, mainly because shaving was so difficult, and almost impossible, with such erratic sight.

I was always delighted to see Dolly, our matron; Shane, my male minder, a perennial presence in Beaumont for me; all the nurses who cared for me, and Professor Eóin O'Brien and his student staff. They were all learning from maestro O'Brien, who was like a wise old tom cat lecturing a posse of acolytes around him. Top Cat!

As life settled into its own routine, every day almost the same, my shadow kept most major concerns at bay, only allowing small niggles to break through the invisible barrier. Things like scans were beginning to register on my awakening mind, together with gym work and going home for the day. While they seem almost mundane now, they assumed enormous proportions then, looming over me like mountains:

> The shadows now so long do grow
> That brambles, like tall cedars grow,
> Molehills seem mountains, and the ant
> Appears a monstrous elephant.

Charles Cotton, 'Evening Quatrains', 1689

Wasn't Charles Cotton quite right? Did he have a brain haemorrhage too? So how else could he describe things so succinctly? It must have been his fertile imagination then, for he was unerringly right.

The first time as a passenger in my wheelchair was a new experience, even a pleasure; there *was* another world after all outside my room; people continually going to and fro, like commuters in a busy railway station. I passed lifts, shops, cafés

and desks, doors, corridors and students, looking self-important with their stethoscopes and white coats. Bless my cynical mind! It was a huge hospital, a pocket mirror of life on the outside.

I was wheeled off on a visit to the hospital ophthalmologist; her surname was new to me but she looked the image of her mother, Corinne, who had been a young student with me in our first year in the College of Science at University College (now government buildings) many years earlier. She told me that my eyes would get progressively better, which eased my mind considerably and shaved kilos from my shadow.

At last I started seeing that slimming shape a bit clearer and I could now begin to look forward. Corinne's daughter was right: my sight began to improve. That was one mini-intruder consigned to its crematorium; another pothole crossed, painlessly.

The next hurdle to take over my prone-to-suggestion mind was a brain scan. I was placed on a conveyor-belt-like contraption and moved into position for this incredible machine to take pictures of my brain, as it clicked in microscopic increments recording my synapses, glial cells and blood vessels, and the odd bit of grey matter presumably mixed up with all that white stuff.

A few days later, while my imagination still played tricks on me, prompting many 'what-ifs' to form and proceed unchallenged, a specialist visited me and consulted the resulting brain photographs. 'Did you ever drink?' he said, sensing a skeleton.

'Until the minute I came in here,' I replied.

'You used to smoke, too,' he said, as if he was omniscient.

'Not since 1982,' I said, feeling as smug as he appeared to be. I waited breathlessly for him, almost expecting him to tell me that I had suffered a subarachnoid haemorrhage; I'm afraid I would have brained him.

But that was another bubble punctured; I now had two back to back. At least my brain scan had shown up nothing abnormal.

My shadow was losing weight rapidly – like myself. I had shed about five stone from the massive twenty or so I'd been carrying around before the event.

I was winning at *something*!

I never fancied the gym in Beaumont; I always found it an almost inhospitable place. It had many familiar objects but the physical routine was difficult and struck me as irrelevant. Perhaps I just wasn't ready.

My first visit there was like taking an escalator to hell; I was wheeled down to this Dungeon of Despair every morning at about 9.30 a.m.; there, I was met by a couple of extremely pleasant, professional-looking female physios and put through many faltering paces. I cannot remember very much, other than my disaffection at the routine daily exercises.

Getting back into my wheelchair after an apparently eventless half-hour, I used to queue along with the others, in our wheelchairs, as my erstwhile helpers clocked in their times and their patients' names at the office, all within earshot of us patients!

My wheelchair driver had me back in my room by about 10.30 a.m. I lay in bed for the remainder of each day with little to do and no way of doing it; frustration and futility made me feel almost useless. This incompatibility with the rehabilitation gymnasium in Beaumont was one shadow that stayed with me until I left for the Rehab Hospital a few weeks later. I felt at that time that I would have been much better off at home, doing exercises throughout the day on my own. There might have been more point to them there; perhaps the thought of the irrational.

Even in my delicate state at the beginning of my recovery I was still dismayed, unsettled by the unnecessary procedure every time I finished my gym work. Obviously people must be paid for what they do, but accounting in detail for their activities, in full hearing of their patients, is both demeaning and insulting to human beings. We may not yet have possessed all our senses, but we were most certainly not a collection of heedless vegetables.

I have no doubt either that a lot of gifted medical and paramedical people ply their trade in that hospital, but I certainly felt that the public relations of the staff as a whole left a lot to be desired and created a sour taste, which still possibly persists, with some patients and their relatives – particularly the relatives. This public relations area is one that needs urgent attention and the criticisms and worries of patients must be attended to promptly and properly. A sort of Parent–Teacher Association to correlate all activities needs to be set up where the patients and their carers can meet the medical staff as equals.

It appears that many medics feel that once surgery is completed successfully, then their job is finished. In fact, that's only one step, albeit a critical one. The major hurdle, once survival ensues, actually is 'What happens next?' for both the family and the patient. Repair and recovery demand the balance of the mental with the physical and have now become major items.

I would never let anyone speak for me; I always made my own mistakes and so could blame nobody else if . . . But it always amazes me that so many otherwise great doctors keep themselves so distant from their patients. In any other profession, most definitely in mine as a vet, they wouldn't get away with it. Medicine can thus seem like a necessary evil, but it shouldn't be; the positive aspects should outshine any negative ones. After all, we are all human, we all make mistakes, unless we're dead.

Plus ça change, plus c'est la même chose! After about seven or eight weeks of protective custody in Beaumont, I was allowed to go home one Saturday, just for the day. I had to be back that night, just like in boarding-school days. It was something to do with keeping a professional eye on me, or because of insurance concerns, or both.

There was much obvious conferring among the staff as I left the cocoon-like safety of the hospital, armed with a list of instructions concerning my well-being and a supply of tablets for almost every contingency. I wouldn't have been surprised if a few contraceptive pills had appeared among the whole pharmacy of drugs, just in case I became pregnant.

However, I truly appreciated all the concerns of the medical staff for my safety, but I did feel a bit like a prize oddity. I was touched that people did care about me and I worked hard to ensure that I wouldn't make a mess of things. But I felt thoroughly incomplete and very dependent.

Anyway, by the time Mandy and Emma arrived for me, I had been dressed for hours. It felt peculiar to have my wife pushing my wheelchair to the car as I allowed myself to be bundled into the front passenger seat, trussed up like a chicken. I was happy to be changing the scenery even for part of a day, and excited to be going home. It was another positive sign of progress, even though I knew full well that the umbilical cord of the car always stayed within shouting distance of the main body back in Beaumont. The car phone added to the feeling of security.

On the way home, which took the best part of an hour, I travelled by many old familiar routes, except this time as a passenger; it was to be for only one of the few times in my adult life, unless I had been under the 'affluence of incohol' and couldn't be trusted to drive safely.

All the recognisable landmarks were still recognisable, but without my specs I saw things in multiple: the cars and trucks and bicycles almost crashed into each other, missed our car by inches and appeared in the most ridiculous, unlikely places – like up a lamp post, on top of a wall or travelling five abreast, with a bus thrown in to make things even more interesting, frightening any complacency out of the oncoming traffic, or so I thought. I eventually shut my eyes and let them do what they wanted. Why should I worry? They could see better than me.

The weather on that first Saturday at home was pleasantly fine, but that didn't really register; just being around, and alive, was of far more significance to me at that incredibly vulnerable stage. I was acutely aware, though, no matter how glad I was to be here on this earth, of the severe limitations of my present condition. Now that I couldn't walk, I certainly felt radically changed, somewhat like a free-flying butterfly forced to undergo reverse metamorphosis, turning back into an earthbound caterpillar again.

I was that lowly caterpillar, though far less mobile, rooted to terra firma and living a mundane, compromised life. How I envied that carefree butterfly, as it hovered noiselessly and effortlessly over the earth, or took wing, athletically flying hither and thither as the whim dictated. How I coveted its helicopter-like abilities! I even envied the caterpillar.

It was always a problem getting the wheelchair in and out of the car, even though it folded up. I doubt if the BMW engineers ever designed a 3-Series coupé to take a wheelchair!

Most things about home were the same; Mandy had had new carpets fitted while I was away, but otherwise everything was in the same place. The dogs were delighted to see me, all claiming me for themselves, almost fighting over me. I never remembered six women fighting over me before. The only other male, Rommel the Alsatian, was delirious. I was equally delighted to see them all again. Mandy and Emma helped me from the car and laid me down on the couch in the lounge; I wasn't yet able to sit in a chair.

Everything seemed familiar, but at the same time the lack of mobility was bizarre. While I was delighted to be around, I found it distressing to be confined so much, whereby my movements were either hugely curtailed or else impossible. I felt useless and foolish, very restricted in what I could do, like in a straitjacket. I had really fallen a long way down, but I had survived, miraculously to most people, and to me; I was now trying to make my way back, claw myself to freedom and safety, inch by painful inch.

I rested and slept on and off during the afternoon, ate some lunch and pretty soon I was back in hospital. I was glad the day had gone without mishap and that I had survived my first taste of freedom. While I was glad to be back in bed, the day at home gave me an appetite for more.

I was glad that I hadn't let Mandy and Emma down and I felt thoroughly grateful to them for all they had done for me. It was an overwhelming feeling to have them caring for me, putting their own lives on hold while they concentrated on my welfare; together with Andrew, they were always unselfish, as they had been right through the brain-haemorrhage episode, and I knew for sure that this would play a monumental part in my rehabilitation.

My goal for now, though, was quite clear: I wanted to be back in Sherlockstown as quickly as possible. My visit home had acted as a prompt. The wait didn't really matter – provided it wasn't too long.

The strident voice was as incisive as a pistol-shot and just as penetrating: 'Pull yourself together, you big shite; you're letting us all down,' he shouted. Shakily recovering from a stagger against the wall, I straightened up in a hurry, resuming my uncertain gait, and looked sheepishly back at the familiar figure of Shane. He was clearly anxious that I should present myself in the best possible light, to convince people that I was better than I actually was. How I was able to walk is still a mystery.

Dr Patrick Murray and I had been in the corridor just outside my room in Caffrey's Ward, trying to establish whether I was capable of making the next move to the National Rehabilitation Hospital in Dún Laoghaire. He had gone to make a phone call, leaving me to contemplate my fragile situation.

ZERO POINT ONE SIX

But Shane's admonition helped to steel my bearing, like sucking in your stomach just long enough for a photograph. Luckily though, I had passed the first test and the Man from Del Monte had said yes; that vote of confidence had been of profound significance to me then, giving me new hope and a fresh focus. I was going to make it.

Overjoyed that the Director of the Rehabilitation Hospital had agreed to accept me as a suitable candidate, I was due to transfer there in about a week. I felt confident and happy to be going onwards. I was obviously worth it; like the girls who use L'Oréal!

At least, I felt, I was progressing to the next stage along the new pathway, but I was still extremely reluctant to leave the familiar safety of Beaumont, which had become like a womb to me. The fears about the proposed move had finally coalesced into a major worry, which felt like the size of a mountain peak. In the days before I left, I heard so much about how the Rehabilitation Hospital differed from Beaumont, how much smaller it was and how like a boot camp the whole place seemed, in direct comparison to a modern, smooth-running major hospital. I remember numerous suggestions that I could expect an institution, rather than a hospital, so different from it and so much less personal than my present oasis; they filled me with foreboding and a desire almost not to go. But this was free will, and anyway I felt ready for far more stimulation than I had experienced during the past weeks of apparently slow progress.

Thinking back on that period now, there is little doubt that the reports that I had heard about the Rehab Hospital, all sounding so negative to my fragile mind, and the almost reluctant admission that it had achieved excellent results, preyed heavily on me, filling me with myriad second thoughts. Bad news and good news.

At the time, all these frightening emotions resulted in weird dreams, more like nightmares, of row upon row of tents, boots of every shape and size all over the kip, exhausted 'prisoners', baying guard dogs, snarling under the barest control of whip-wielding Kapos: those guards picked from among the prisoners themselves, there just to keep the poor, suffering inmates from escaping.

I often woke up suddenly in the days just before my departure, soaked with sweat and anxious with fear. The feeling still plagues me that I should have been far better prepared for taking the huge next step along the uncertain route to rehabilitation and recovery; not frightened out of my wits.

As that marvellous book *The Diving Bell and the Butterfly*, by the now-deceased Frenchman Jean-Dominique Bauby, told us, people who have lost the power of speech are often still fully capable of hearing. He had; he was. I was almost the opposite: able to see, speak and hear but, unlike Bauby, *not* capable of handling the negative aspects of where I was going.

It was unbelievably motivating that the author dictated the text by blinking his eyelids to convey the exact letters from the alphabet to his interpreter. Amazing. I know now for certain that it does not stretch the intelligence of anyone too much to concede that detailed descriptions, no matter how well meaning, must be properly dressed up for certain patients, who, like me, were numbed by doubt and worry.

I now know, because I found out the hard way, that after a major mishap in one's life, a serious setback, when one is making excellent but still rather painful progress, many patients often look far better than they physically or mentally feel. In my case (perhaps a lively imagination was the root cause of my heightened concerns), these worries, which another patient might cast aside as of little consequence, bothered me immensely. This experience greatly influenced me, colouring my view at the time and causing me no end of anxiety: it was a heavy weight on my mind.

Hindsight, being a brilliant prognostician, where facts are rarely wrong, suggests that psychologists or psychotherapists should be employed by all hospitals; their job description would be to introduce recovering patients like me gradually to major changes like the one I was about to undertake. It *was* a glaring omission to leave such important details in the hands of the nursing staff, who were not experienced at presenting such places or events to patients like myself, certainly not as a psychologist would have been able to do, and whose specialities, no matter how appropriate to sick beds, did not extend to the labyrinths of the mind.

Anyway, having said my reluctant goodbyes to Dolly, Shane and the nurses who had cared for me so superbly, I was wheeled in an ambulance trolley to the rear entrance of the hospital. It was probably only a few minutes, but that journey felt like an age and the pangs of pain on leaving were something like seeing your infant quit the warmth of your bed for the progress of the cot; irrespective of how normal, it is always a painful experience.

I was strapped into the trolley bed on the waiting Waverly ambulance, and as we drove away a large lump formed in my throat, tears misted my eyes and my gut was in turmoil from a vice of steel. I felt awful. It was with the heaviest of hearts that I bade adieu to dear old Beaumont, home for so many weeks, as I began the long journey across the city and the next major adventure in my new life. I missed Mandy, Emma and Andrew to an incredible degree, they had been always with me up until now. My older daughters, Sharon and Amanda, would hear about all my movements from Andrew, and they too would now feel able to visit me more often in the Rehab; the hospital atmosphere in Beaumont didn't entice them to overvisit me there. The smell of disinfectant and that peculiar hospital aroma did not agree with them. My head was in a hopeless jumble. I felt lost and alone, and afraid, for the very first time in my life. I was a very dependent patient.

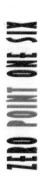

FIVE

Back to Basics

When I eventually left Beaumont for the Rehabilitation Hospital I had undergone a transformation, whereby my shadow changed its outline from a survival mode to a more repair and recovery orientated one. Going off to Dún Laoghaire represented the start of a new life for me, and it would be a slimmer, fitter shadow that came with me. It now kept pace beside me. I had obviously stayed long enough under the overpowering umbrella of my own purgatory and was looking forward to escaping.

The journey to Dún Laoghaire felt an interminably long one, which it wasn't. After the first fifty yards or so, I could have been walking on Mars or motoring on the moon: I had as much clue where I was as a captive dumped in a car trunk. The jingle of coins at some point during the trip told me we had crossed the Liffey at the East Link toll-bridge. Otherwise I was lost, trying to envisage our route in my mind's eye – like a jailed inmate playing mental chess – but I gave up. I just couldn't concentrate.

I had begun this trip with a lot of trepidation about my intended stay in the Rehab Hospital, remembering all those adverse things that had been said about the place: like how difficult it would be to conform to the restrictive regime there. I wanted to make progress and get better (did I what?), but I didn't

ZERO POINT ONE SIX

fancy the thought of going through all the trials particular to a military-style environment: plenty of pain and debatable gain. But I must have been daft or off in Utopia to have expected little hardship.

Eventually we arrived and I was wheelchaired into a plain but pleasant single room facing the front, on the first floor. The place seemed friendly, warm and welcoming. Things began to look good from the very first minute, prompting thoughts that I was going to like it here.

I sat in my room, reflecting on the many changes in my life, having put my bits and pieces away in lockers, like a back packer in a youth hostel.

Then, when I was helping to fill out the entry form the lady in charge of admissions asked me a seemingly innocuous question: 'What's your ambition in here, Michael?'

'To get the hell out of this place as fast as I can,' I said, meaning no disrespect to my new abode or its staff.

Having established my routine, I handed over my hymn sheet of rules and discussed whatever medication I was taking.

Before I began the recovery programme proper, I had a day to settle in, poking around like a lost visitor, trying to become familiar with the nooks and crannies. Luckily for me, my cousin Liam Dennehy was also a guest of the Rehab, arriving weeks before me; he was an 'old hand' by now, having been admitted with the after-effects of a stroke. We had grown up together in Currow, a little village in County Kerry, knowing most things about each other. He was a few years younger than me; his brother Hugh, my friend also, just one year older. Liam and his girlfriend Julie married and had a family; he worked at the Agriculture Institute in Grange, County Meath, about twenty miles from Dublin. He was always such a fit and health-conscious bloke that I was highly surprised when he suffered a stroke; shocked to see him incapacitated.

But I was grateful at the same time that he could show me the ropes and allay my many worries, since our roles were now reversed; he had had his stroke at a time when I felt normal. My incident post-dated his by a couple of months. In a perverse sort of way, I was glad of his company in such a strange place.

Cousins Margaret and Helen, Liam's sisters, visited me a few times in Beaumont, representing, as it did, another strongish thread stretching towards a return to reality for me, and I greeted them with all the joy I felt at being able even to see them again. Words can barely describe the incredible feeling of warmth and hope at meeting your close family, particularly when you'd thought you'd never see them again, when you were in the worst possible shape of your life.

Our other cousin Maureen was a regular visitor whom I was always delighted to see. In the early days in Beaumont she observed, 'Gosh, Mick, it's great to see you; you'll make it back perfect, won't you?'

'I hope so,' I said, the emphasis on the 'hope'.

'When you start back writing again, you can say "I'll be a changed boy from now on, I won't ever again write anything controversial!"' As if I ever would.

Anyway, I retorted, 'Maureen, you know I'm not that badly affected in the brain department. I'll get back into print OK, but then I'll say "You ain't seen nothing yet!"' I never did though.

However, Margaret and Helen, Maureen and Julie became regular visitors during my time in the Rehab Hospital, and they helped make all the struggles worth the effort.

Thankfully, nothing looked even vaguely similar to what I had been led to expect. I had had visions, for example, of some kind of concentration camp, but I didn't notice anybody going around in prison garb. There were no guards, no bars on the windows or doors, and not a sign of potential escapees hiding furtively in bushes, waiting for the safety cover of darkness. I was cautiously relieved. So far, so good.

Obviously those who had been putting the frighteners on me back in Beaumont, perhaps thinking that they were doing me a favour, had it all wrong. It was something like those newspaper

film critics when I was a university student; having found out early on that their tastes and mine did not exactly synchronise, I never bothered reading them again, depending instead on my own instincts. Generally I was right and far more in tune with my personal likes and dislikes. But life now in my new state was no mere movie; it was harsh reality, very definitely make-your-mind-up time, as I was about to find out.

Suddenly I missed the whole support system of Beaumont Hospital: Professor O'Brien, Dolly, Shane, all the nurses who looked after me, in Intensive and Coronary Care, and the wheel-chair-porters, all seemed such a distant memory, a pleasant interlude that felt as if it was in another life, disjointed from the present.

The routine of being pushed everywhere in wheelchairs wasn't going to happen in Dún Laoghaire; I had to learn to push my own wheels. There seemed to be an acute shortage of porters; I definitely didn't see any of them loitering about, smoking fags and scratching their backsides, just awaiting my pleasure, like bored taxi-drivers.

The headlines in this place screamed out loud and clear: 'The Lord helps those who help themselves.' Any kind of mollycoddling was for the post-surgical after-care of Beaumont, and very definitely all ties with the lifestyle there had been abruptly severed; there was to be no going back. It was like pulling out the plug of a television set. Finality. Surgery was over. Now survival had become the first stage on the road to recovery.

I had to learn many new names and new faces all over again. Having met the key people in the various departments, I found that the whole place exuded the life of a new and friendly society. It was nothing like the boot camp I had envisaged, more like a holiday camp, where residents, sporting various disabilities, were being helped to cope, to shake off their infirmities and face the big bad world again.

In Dún Laoghaire, even at a cursory glance, the aura of self-help and acceptance sprouted everywhere, like a mission statement; instead of being pampered, the patients were encouraged to look after themselves, more or less. In fact, the term 'patient' did not quite seem to fit at all; the friendly faces proclaimed that their owners were more like guests, all obviously happy to be here, despite the unfortunate circumstances.

If driving your own wheelchair was a giant step, learning to walk again was a long jump. There was obviously a certain amount of passive activity, like sitting and freewheeling, involved in wheelchairing, but absolutely nil in walking. I now know exactly how Neil Armstrong felt, taking that 'first small step for man' and 'the giant leap for mankind' on the moon all those years before. He couldn't have put it better.

To get around the compact Rehab Hospital, I had to have wheels powered all by myself. After a shaky start, becoming accustomed to all this newness of not being pushed, I quickly got into the swing; I learned from watching the others in wheelchairs, who screamed past me with apparent ease, that working your feet alone, actually walking along the ground, instead of using your arms to propel the wheels, speeded things up considerably, and also conserved one's meagre strength. Ingenuity was clearly alive and well.

By degrees, I became an experienced old hand at the wheels, but I was a very reluctant driver. I would have preferred to have been able to walk. Years earlier I had heard the blind Lenny Peters, of Peters and Lee 1970s' fame, being interviewed on BBC Radio by some twit, about losing his eyesight in an accident with guitar strings (I think). 'You'd probably prefer being blind now, Lenny, with all this high-profile stuff with your songs, rather than still having your eyesight, but remaining a "nobody",' said the crass interviewer.

ZERO POINT ONE SIX

'You must be bloody jokin', mate,' an outraged Lenny replied.

Ken Ging friend from Bray, County Wicklow, took a photo of me during a visit. I was sitting relaxed, soaking up the late summer sun, with my empty wheelchair lying discarded and forlorn beside a garden seat. The caption on the back simply read 'to hell with the wheelchair'. It captured my feelings exactly, a bit like Neil Armstrong, but different. Ken and I were both glad to meet again; we had known each other as players and again when we both became involved with Leinster. We shared great memories.

That ageing wheelchair, though, was both a blessing and a provocation; it was always with me, acting as a powerful motivating influence, and I needed every scrap of stimulation. It served as a constant reminder that a challenge always waited for me.

But much as I dreamed about the future or rode along on the horseback of make-believe, I had to be content for the moment with the exciting prospect of 'upgrading' to a Zimmer frame and the invalid's aluminium walking-stick. Who the hell was Zimmer anyway? An invalid? Probably Doctor Wolfgang Zimmer, orthopaedic surgeon über alles.

I was truly amazed at the different types of residents in the Rehab Hospital, the extent of their infirmities and the number of people I had recognised there. They were from nearly all walks of life and all age-groups. Their disabilities ranged from no arms at all, to one arm or one leg, differing degrees of paralysis, poor speech, no speech and rickety balance. I felt particular empathy with the few people whom I knew (and vice versa) who could not speak at all, despite showing full recognition and a terrific longing to talk. It must have been incredibly difficult for them to handle, and it was terribly moving.

Tom 'Skib' O'Driscoll had qualified as a vet with me years earlier; we both immediately recognised each other, silently sympathising with our respective conditions by our shared looks of unasked questions, but even though we wanted to talk, we couldn't. His speech had been removed by a stroke. Life is often cruel, always indiscriminate.

In the hospital one could see the greatest concentration of physically compromised people that one could imagine in any one place. The mind marvelled at the extent of it all – at least mine did. It was a salutary experience to be suddenly confronted by hospital wards filled with those who were flawed but alive, who had survived various life-threatening episodes, wanting desperately to get better, and to that end would subject themselves to almost any regime. I had no doubt that necessity was the mother of invention, and the father as well.

It was very gratifying to observe the ever-friendly staff demonstrating the qualities of care and concern, which one could have written to Santa for, and to see the immediate families displaying support for their less fortunate relatives, or best friends, who had been so cruelly cut down.

It was enlightening to realise that while all patients were expected to work hard at their own salvation, the full support of staff and relatives was extremely important; crucial even. The fact that all the principal actors in this human drama were rowing towards the same finishing line, in complete synchronicity, added enormously to the expected outcome. Families were vital, and I never once saw staff members lose their patience – despite frequent provocation.

What occurred to me most forcibly, once again, was the surprise, even the shock in some instances, that so many previously normal people had finished up in this Rehab Hospital. It was extremely humbling when you first experienced the true extent of people's suffering in a so-called civilised society – before they ever came to this Last Chance Saloon. I still feel that way, and during the many stages of my own tenancy in the Rehab Hospital I was filled with wonder at their quiet acceptance of their new infirmities, and amazed at the extent of their resolve to improve their circumstances. It was astonishingly uplifting.

In stark contrast, my own deficiencies, though life-threatening

ZERO POINT ONE SIX

at the beginning, felt almost minuscule by comparison and far less long term. My rapidly sobering perspective suffered a further shake-up during the initial assessment in the Physiotherapy Department.

In this hallowed hall, any wheelchair-assisted camouflaging is stripped away, as by a lover's lingering look, when these physios put you through your paces, revealing all the candid physical details that you would prefer not to show. Everyone else who could be bothered can see too. There is no hiding place in the Physio Department.

I asked my assessor, the recently qualified John Murphy from Newmarket, County Cork, how he handled such an array of maladies. He replied confidently in his laid-back manner, 'We're actually trained to work with most conditions and most situations, so we become very accustomed to coping quite quickly.' I could appreciate all that. 'But, Mick,' said he, in all seriousness, 'you are lucky to be starting out yourself at a point where many people here will probably finish up. They may not get much more appreciably better, even after quite a few months; but you can. It's up to you.' I considered myself lucky.

Perceptions, of course, are always relative: what some patients feel is enormous progress to them may not seem of such importance to able-bodied people. It certainly ensured, though, that I didn't let any opinions of myself reach dizzying heights; but simultaneously I didn't need much arm-twisting to get better. I got the distinct impression that self-opinionated people would be as conspicuous here as white bodies among a colony of sun-worshippers.

The surprise of being confronted with stark reality, and having to face up to the extent of my own disabilities (not measuring them against anybody else's, but looking at them in direct contrast to the way I used to be, even if I usually did most things to excess), came as a real shaft of realism to me; but there were even more surprises in store.

One day, about to buzz off on my chariot of painfully slow wheels to my room, to relax after the morning's exertions, I said to John Murphy: 'By the way, John, when people appear through the door for the first time, and you don't know anything much about them personally, how do you decide whether they'll make it or not?'

Quick as a flash he shot back, 'Good question, Mick, but I see only winners and losers.' Touché. I had been half-expecting some intelligent-sounding mumbo-jumbo about the psychology of purposeful intent becoming wedded with the physical benefits of various exercise programmes, propelling physical incompletes on to new stages of quest and achievement, like mountain climbers or motivation lectures (I know, I've given enough of them, too): 'I climbed that mountain just because it was there' or 'How I did it in ten easy lessons'. Like the singer Val Doonican, who claimed that he became an overnight success, but, in fact, it took him thirty years!

But I was wrong about long-winded motivation-speak. Winners and losers – nothing else. John Murphy was right, of course, and he certainly changed my life. Pretence was consigned to the dustbin, and I began to look for winners everywhere I could. I felt that my detection work revealed an odd loser, but, thankfully, there were nearly all winners in Dún Laoghaire.

But, from the perspective of the assessors, and the physiotherapy helpers, with their all-seeing laser eyes, the motivation sessions of all modern sports groups must appear to be a whole industry; it boils down, of course, in the end to winners and losers.

All life does, too. You must really *want* something, *crave* something badly enough, right from the very beginning. As Bill Shankley of Liverpool Football Club once said, long ago, 'Winning isn't everything; it's the only thing.' An infamous US coach also observed that 'Ninety-five per cent of my income goes on wine, women and song; I just squander the rest of it.' I knew exactly how he felt.

I was extremely fortunate to have had John Murphy as my first teacher in the Rehab Hospital; he started me on the rocky road to recovery. If I didn't improve it would be my own fault; I couldn't blame him. Luckily for me he was a superb teacher. I knew it at the time, but I certainly appreciate it now.

When I was in secondary school in Newbridge College, in the 1950s, our mathematics teacher, Tim Ryan, would recite this ditty regularly:

> Big fleas have little fleas
> Upon their backs to bite 'em;
> Little fleas have smaller fleas
> And so ad infinitum.

I never knew exactly why at the time, but now many years later it has taken on a mantle of realism. We never looked anything like fleas, but the demons which accompanied most of us could be symbolised as such minuscule menaces, metaphorically speaking of course. Though small in stature, these little demonic pests varied in size, like humans, from the fat to the skinny, but were still present in sufficient numbers to cause many problems. There is a danger in numbers, too, and size *doesn't* really matter, either. But my shadowy demons took on the shape of fleas, always threatening.

After their initial assessment, I assumed that the technical staff had drawn up a clearer picture of my physical and mental state, a sort of baseline from which we could all proceed.

I encountered many familiar faces on my first work-day at the gym; in fact I was relieved and delighted to see so many people I knew, and so I readily acknowledged their friendly greetings.

The self-consciousness I felt while trundling along in my wheelchair, and my still feeble capacity for moving around unaided, all cleared away gradually like a smoke-filled room does when a window is opened. I could see clearly that this gymnasium was a true layby for broken bodies and psychologically battered souls, both in urgent need of fixing.

How these two parts of us had become so inextricably dependent on each other, linked like love knots, was remarkable, but not unexpected; this was to become more and more relevant as day succeeded day, but it is safe to assume that most people started out on their recovery paths armed only with positive mental and physical attitudes, liberally sprinkled with cautious optimism. They were ready for anything.

The gym was a large fresh-smelling room, purpose-built to accommodate oodles of activities, all seemingly happening simultaneously. It was at least 150 feet long by 60 feet wide – I know, I either wheelchaired or staggered nearly every painful square foot of it. I don't know how high the ceiling was (I never got to that stage), but it was very airy, lending an aura of spaciousness. There were large windows all along its left side, which overlooked the rear of the carpark and the grounds beyond – almost another country.

When you came in the front door, usually in your wheelchair, the atmosphere conveyed a hive of relatively silent industry – like a hand-weaving carpet factory I once visited in Morocco. Down the right-hand side of the room were five or six exercise beds, with curtains to screen off prying eyes and to allow some privacy. In the centre of the floor were various large exercise mats, boxes of assorted rubber balls, some quite large. At one end of the gymnasium were exercise bicycles, wall-fixed weights, special tables for arm and hand exercises and a few exercise bunks occupied the other. Exercise was infectious.

Two long walking-frames, like the more usual parallel bars in a gym, took up most of the left-hand side, extending from a set

ZERO POINT ONE SIX

of stairs (to practise going up and coming down – the 'Grand Old Duke of York' routine) on the back wall, right up to the imposing-looking clock on the other. This maestro of time looked in surprisingly pristine condition; it was a clean off-white colour, despite all the glances of frustration, irritation, botheration, expectation, exhaustion, and, oh yes, gratitude – sentiments that were all regularly thrown its way. In the early days, I couldn't make out what time its hands said, but soon I was fitted with my first set of spectacles since that 14 July 'happening'. The miracle of improved sight greatly encouraged me.

If you can envisage it, there was ample space on either side of the central mats for various athletic activities. All the spaces were occupied by bruised bodies hard at work, with a physio alternating between groups of two or three people. There were wheelchairs lying about, like an invalids' convention, or a day out at the seaside; the chairs were either moving around as if they were on roller blades, or else lying abandoned, patiently waiting for their owners to return – like faithful pets. They would all have been wheel-clamped out on the street!

Everyone looked busy and, no matter how strenuous or easy any particular activity might seem to the casual observer, in full possession of their intact faculties, I knew only too well the blood, sweat and tears, the determination and the incredible will-power that accompanied even the most mundane-looking efforts. One person would be lifting leg weights; others might be learning how to regain their balance, using only their stomach muscles on medicine balls (and I thought only boxers or fitness fanatics did that); still others would be proceeding to take their first, slow, painful steps along the hand-assisted walkways – probably their first attempts at walking for many months. They had all begun to recognise the full import of their plights and were coming to terms with the insults to their bodies, bodies that would never be quite the same again.

As a well-known friend, who used to live in Pittsburgh, said to me once, quite early on when I was in the recovering-at-home phase, 'Mick, we'll never again play against England on a wet afternoon.' We were too old anyway, but I knew exactly what he meant. Changed forever.

Tony O'Reilly, the then head of the global Heinz Corporation, also had a seismic effect on my recovery at this crucial time: I was sitting at home, contemplating no higher than my navel and feeling sorry for myself, when Tony phoned from the States. His simplicity galvanised me, making me realise that I must accept my present lot, get off my butt and aim for the nearest stars again. A push I badly needed.

Tony was undoubtedly, by far, the foremost International Rugby player of his era; he remains one of the most accomplished people I have ever met. He has been knighted recently, now known as Sir Anthony, in rightful recognition of his enviable profile, especially his work over the years with the Ireland Fund (All Ireland). To many of us, though, he'll always be the 'Bould Reilly'; we don't actually need the title to remind us of one of nature's one-offs. Anyway his words helped me immeasurably.

Some people found that the actual walking wasn't too difficult; instead, they had to relearn to do the simplest hand and finger exercises, with the aid of electronic machines. The stiffness of their fingers, which were reluctant to budge, made each movement an agony – the agony and frustration that one can experience only when old, familiar actions have been shut down, closed up with inactivity for stagnant months and were now being coaxed back into working order again displaying all the reluctance of a stubborn pet.

Every few hours a new band of aspirants arrived, and the tired bodies who had been hard at work went off about their other business until their afternoon sessions. The new arrivals took

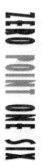

their places, going through their routines like old hands, which many of them were. Familiarity bred confidence and a sort of warm content. Never contempt.

Personally, I found that riding on the exercise bike and doing the various leg exercises prescribed for me became gradually easier after a few weeks, but all attempts at walking, even a few wobbly steps, seemed like a marathon. My brain and my legs seemed as if they had never been introduced.

There was little doubt that this establishment was a highly organised rehabilitation hospital, geared towards the most focused procedures and programmes possible, to help one get better; in some instances I would say I had little choice – I was being wafted along on a favourable wind with its own driving force.

Beaumont Hospital seemed a long time ago; it was a general hospital, geared more to treatment surgery and survival, while the National Rehab was dedicated specifically to rehabilitation, treatment, repair and recovery. I was glad to be alive and able to assist my helpers. I could certainly thank Beaumont for that. Were it not for everything about the place, and everyone working and living there, I would have been dead and buried by now.

Anyway, I spent that first day at the gym – an hour in the morning, another after lunch – doing all the exercises that I could do on my front and on my back, except for the obvious ones! Once I had become accustomed to raising my now spindly legs up and down, singly or together and repeating the procedures on my front, leg weights up to five kilos each were then introduced to the schedule fairly promptly, to add the extra resistance to my rapidly tiring muscles.

I also learned how to do various things to strengthen my flabby stomach muscles, to prepare me for eventual walking. 'Things' correctly describes my efforts; 'exercises' sound a little too much like co-ordination.

After about a week of this daily toil, I was cured of my

anticipation of 'easie peasie' or of being tempted by the cockiness of familiarity! However, without ever becoming self-satisfied, I did feel that I was definitely making progress: my muscles were becoming that bit stronger and my mind more and more at ease, more focused on the long distant end. I reckoned that I could eventually make it if I tried hard enough. The gym had become central to everything in my recovery.

There was roughly an equal split between the sexes, even though I had always equated bodily insults like strokes with males. And I doubt if the tantalising mating ritual of butterflies flitted across anybody's mind in Dún Laoghaire; certainly not mine, and Viagra tablets would probably have lain around in full view, rapidly deteriorating, like overripe bananas or half-rotten apples. Walking was more relevant than love-making. For the time being anyway.

I was fascinated and impressed by the atmosphere that pervaded the whole hospital; anywhere patients congregated was dominated by a definite agenda which appeared everywhere like a menu; the whole place oozed getting better. It was obvious, even to the visitor, that while our infirmities might be personal, there existed almost an overwhelming air of sharing, a true community spirit. It was as if a statement had been hung on the entrance door, simply announcing, 'You don't come here for holidays; the purpose of your visit is to get better.'

The purpose and enthusiasm that almost everyone displayed created a wholly positive atmosphere, the like of which you'd find around a good team that knew exactly what it was about; all activities looked well planned and synchronised – they had to be or else chaos would reign. Straightaway I knew that all my activities had been well orchestrated and proven in advance and I had very little chance of mitching from school!

When you ponder about it, it must be relatively easy to

ZERO POINT ONE SIX

maintain enthusiasm about something when the expected results take only a limited, defined time span to achieve; however, when landmines of uncertainty litter the journey, turning it into an awkward obstacle course, things necessarily become far more difficult.

The motivating drive to become whole again, to maintain the right attitude towards improvement, certainly can take a fair old hammering, especially when, after an initial period of promise, the struggle extends into one large, never-ending slog. It then becomes extremely difficult for everyone.

It is exactly at this point though, that the cleft-stick syndrome takes over, exploiting even the slightest opportunity. The *long haul*, depending on an ending that stretches off to the distant horizon, can dampen even the keenest enthusiasm. That's understandable. But, on the other hand, it is well nigh impossible to make any true progress towards a fairly normal state unless one is charged up like a battery, armed with a strictly positive mindset; and all this, despite the understandable periods of pessimism that can afflict the human psyche from time to time.

But in your eagerness to avoid pitfalls and do the right thing, you cannot rush at things either, like a child in a toyshop. Patience is always a virtue and it requires constant discipline to adhere rigidly to your own physical regimen and to keep firmly focused.

Whatever had occurred during your former lifetime obviously did not matter a damn now; time-scales took on a totally different meaning and we were all encouraged to exorcise from our minds the kinds of people we had previously been; and at the same time, we had to embrace wholeheartedly, even to the point of getting to like, the new individuals that we had to become. Some metamorphosis! But it was central from now on.

Taking your time, in your own good time, was now the predominating phrase – take your time but hurry up! I must admit that I found the lack of group competitiveness, the fact that I had to concentrate on nobody but myself, disorientating at first; all my life, after all, had been centred on taking on somebody, at something. Ah well! Relaxing was obviously in vogue, and moderation probably would have kept me out of there. But now suddenly the competition was restricted to myself and my own infirmities.

The whole process felt like being kitted out with a wholly new personality, or having your persona and former lifestyle peeled away, layer after injured layer by a clever shrink, to be rebuilt from scratch. That's how I saw life now.

Setting definite, realistic goals became the overriding concern of all of us, centrally important when we each faced our daily struggles. If you really think about it, Attila the Hun would have been demotivated himself if he had been faced with a long, indefinite future as well. He, too, couldn't thrive on uncertainty.

At any rate, the obligatory transformation from street civvies into clothes more appropriate to the gym proved relatively easy for most people who had considered how their lives had altered, and what the future promised. As far as I could make out, their conversion to confronting realism was ably abetted by their families and close friends, proving that a stroke, like other afflictions, is a family affair. It was for me anyway. The symbolism of shedding street clothes was also evident to most of us: casting off old identities and embracing a new way of life had become our master key.

Understandably too, many people, especially those with longer lasting infirmities, took extra time to make the necessary mental changes; they were possibly a bit disillusioned, even deflated, by the initial Giant Steps along the recuperation trail that were visibly being made by some of their more fortunate companions.

However, as with most things in life, their perseverance achieved the right goal in the end, and they succeeded in making the most telling readjustments; becoming ready and able to meet the challenges that lay ahead. I have since seen a street poster with the message 'You will fail only when you give up'; it appealed to me with its simplicity, its accuracy.

After the faltering start of the learner, we soon became more aware of our own wants, more tuned in to our lives. The antennae of any alien never bristled so attentively; our receptors were set in ready mode to receive each new signal. We seemed to be saying 'Throw everything you want at us; we can handle it!'

Then, again, you couldn't help noticing that a few people were really struggling, finding their sudden impediments and the mental acceptance of their lot very difficult to take. They appeared to be ignoring the new realities and their futures must have held out little hope for them, as they saw it. They were in obvious need of the most urgent psychological counselling from a trained psychologist, who could help them and their distracted families, to comprehend and accept what had befallen them; a psychologist who could explain their radically altered circumstances, as well as suggesting how they should proceed. We *all* needed a mind-mender.

Personally, I was too introverted at this critical time to even bother with my fellow-patients, much as I could feel their need. I was having enough trouble keeping my own self afloat, but I couldn't help noticing so large a gap in the system – an otherwise excellent one; it was a simple fact that a specialist in psychology, a professional, was needed to fill such a void.

I am sure that the authorities really only want 'winners' to enter the Rehab Hospital, but obviously the odd troubled person gets through the selection process as well, and seemingly cannot help themselves; they are in urgent need of the assistance of a mind-doctor. That is crystal.

The balance between the physical fitness of the body and the mind's unpredictable labyrinth is as vital to a recovering patient as it is to the success of any well-oiled team machine. However, I was faced with looking after my own requirements rather than those of footballers, and I knew how important my own philosophy and mental attitudes were to my progress from invalid to fully functioning human. Self-centredness ruled.

Of course, in this unusual community of impaired limbs and minds there was little that was abnormal or odd. We were all the same, just afflicted in different ways. Some of us had had a stroke whose effects varied in severity; others had suffered different, seriously incapacitating mishaps, while still others, minus their limbs, had to have new replacement hands and legs fitted. We were all brushed by tragedy. Life had certainly 'happened' to us – with a fury!

It struck me, almost being skewered into my consciousness, that all our previous conveyor-belt kinds of living had been overturned in a major way. Almost like a remarriage, we were being given a second chance to get things right, our lives now suddenly a fruit compote, not the unified smooth beings we once were; while our more normal compadres on the outside still only had the one life to be going on with – not many of whom would make the changes that they should, either.

It *was* exciting to realise that we were unique in another way too: *only we*, ourselves, were being given the unequivocal opportunity to begin life anew and select a different direction to before, when high living had probably caused our 'bungee jumping' in the first place.

However, I cannot blame anybody for not radically changing their lifestyles. I might believe that they are misdirected in a potentially dangerous way, but I wouldn't level any blame. I doubt whether I would have chosen a clear-cut alteration in my own lifestyle either, if I hadn't had that fright of a brain

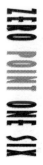

SIX

Childish Dreams

Cats are supposed to have nine lives, such is their uncanny luck. People are deemed to enjoy their second childhood in late adult life, around the time they reach the ripe old age of eighty. On this basis I must be extremely fortunate – I got mine quite soon in my career, around early mid-life, when survival from the unexpected stroke gave me another chance at living. Could I still look forward to a third, later on?

Mandy had already helped me to realise how happy life after divorce could be, making me a more complete person in the process and giving us a beautiful little present in Emma, a sister for Andrew, Sharon and Amanda, children from my first marriage with Lynne. It was therefore with a more than considerable amount of gratitude that I could again enjoy, with unabashed enthusiasm, the family that had almost become past tense for me.

There really wasn't much point in setting up a hammock, relaxing high up among my laurels, while I considered how fortunate I was; I had to get up off my fat bum and prove conclusively that I could grab the opportunities of life again with every hook and fibre of my consciousness.

But the fat lady wasn't about to sing for a long time yet. Just

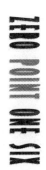

ZERO POINT ONE SIX

because I had made it this far, with most of the effort coming from others, and the prospect still of many more difficult obstacles to negotiate, it didn't imply that she was about to burst into a verse of the 'Hallelujah Chorus' in celebration. Her singing and my improving were critically dependent on each other; and so the celebrations could stay on hold for a while yet.

There *was* a purpose to all the calisthenics and muscle exercises that I had been labouring over in the gym; it meant that I had to begin to walk, whether I liked to or not. But could I? Mentally, I felt that I could, or that I would do so at some stage. Physically I was unsure if I was up to it; I didn't want the spluttering engine to let me down. I felt that whatever progress I would make would be a kind of floodwater mark for many other people too, in their own quest for rehabilitation, and I couldn't disappoint so many expectant minds. We all depended on each other for motivation. I may have been struck down like everybody else, but I felt in my bones that I had to perform. John Murphy had ideas other than just allowing me to take life easy: he wanted me walking as soon as possible. So I was introduced, unfussily, to the dreaded parallel bars.

However, my imagination proved bigger than my appetite; I had bitten off much more than I could munch, and what looked reasonably easy to us, the cognoscenti, from the vantage of cool wheelchairs, or exercise beds, was a different proposition when I had to do it myself. I found it excruciatingly hard.

My hands were guided on to the wooden bars, as if they belonged to someone else, my body was supported, and I was constantly supervised. Even with all the help and encouragement of the staff and the silent good wishes of numerous watching residents, I felt that putting one leg in front of the other was a brand-new experience for me. I'm glad my rugby team-mates and friends did not see me then, reduced to learning to walk all over again. Any comparison between my present plight and international rugby was as ridiculous as trying to roller-skate on sand dunes. It really was no consolation at all that I had ever played for or against anybody – it didn't seem to matter a curse.

On one hand it *was* sad to reflect in my present state on all the training I had done on the track and in the gym at Fenners, Cambridge University's famous cricket ground, sharing sweat and grunts with Ireland's Mike Gibson and Brian Rees of Wales.

The following year, 1967, Brian was consistently misbehaving in the Wales v Ireland game in Cardiff Arms Park, while the poor English referee, flushed with frustration, implored him and his Welsh team-mates to 'observe the laws for God's sake'. It was a waste of time. Eventually in exasperation, the ref, knowing full well that we three were Cambridge colleagues, admonished us with the stern warning, 'If Mr Rees transgresses once more, I'll have to send *all of you guys* off!' And we had done nothing!

Brian was warned in no uncertain terms by us what 'the score was' and, full marks to him, he played on like a saint; if any Welshman ever played like a saint. In a sort of perverse way the fact of having been a senior sportsman at one time began to act as a sort of headline to me, prodding me mentally to get back to some sort of everyday living. It worked in the end.

Anyway, the tendency, the compulsion at this stage was to lose all sense of balance, almost falling over on my front or on to my back, all the while keeping my feet too close together and looking down at my toes. I suppose it was a natural reaction to bewildered uncertainty, but it was incorrect and I had to be constantly reminded, 'Look up. See where you're going', 'Keep your feet wider apart to help your balance' or 'Don't fall over' (as if I'd wanted to!).

Walking between these wooden guiderails, in a straight line, one foot in front of the other, as if I was measuring off the distance in feet, was extremely difficult. It had to be done though, it was a pain, but it was integral to the whole walking experience, far more central to it all than I had ever before imagined.

I thought back to my much younger days, waiting in the queue at the dry cleaner's in Tralee, in County Kerry, and looking

around for something to read, to help pass the time. Ralph Waldo Emerson's words 'Life is not so short but that there is always time for courtesy' have stuck firmly in my mind ever since, but the other framed, stark quotation, high up on the facing wall, which made the more forceful impression, simply stated, 'I once complained about my feet until I met a man with no legs.'

I still had both my legs, albeit temporarily less useful ones, and I couldn't very well complain that all these exercises and attempts at walking were killing me. I had a long way to go; I had the physical assets to make it, no matter how compromised they were at present, and I had to make certain that my mental attitude matched my ambitions. My own afflicted limbs were all I had to rely on, as well as the good wishes of other patients and the determination to make it.

After a while I began to make steady progress at the parallel bars' walking exercises; I learned how to walk with only one hand resting on the bars, then no hands – being ready all the while to grab any support, in case I fell. I became an expert grabber! It felt like being a trainee athlete in a circus, walking a tightrope, with a safety net for security and holding on to a support for reassurance.

I then moved on to balancing exercises, on special wooden rocking boards, while I was kept upright all the while by the parallel bars. It was obviously all geared towards further improving my balance and getting me more accustomed to sensations from my feet, just like vibrations and messages from the road surface are transmitted to your body via the car seats and your bottom. No doubt it was a great routine, but it was really awkward to do. Try it, fully fit, with your eyes shut, with no hands supporting you and I defy most people to do it correctly. I often failed.

Many days later I began walking outside the bars on the gymnasium's wooden floor, gradually letting go of the supporting props (with my hands hovering over the bars, always poised in case I made a blunder). All this activity required the constant attention of the physio in case I fell, which I often did. However, I wasn't on my own. We were all learner drivers in the gym, with our driving tests waiting for us.

Gradually, floppy, fatigued muscles began to harden up, and tasks that had looked preposterous only a short while before had now become part of rehabilitation and recovery; fellow-residents spoke encouraging things, and the uncertain confidence department received a much-needed boost.

I didn't doubt that I would improve, but I didn't know exactly when or how long it would take. Subconsciously I revelled in the support of my fellow-sufferers, my peers, and then everything began to look a bit brighter.

The 'Look straight ahead. Watch where you're going' mantra, continually offered by John Murphy, became so established in my subconscious that it had assumed the importance almost of eating. I even suffered nightmares about it and all his other admonitions, too. I secretly hoped that John Murphy's dreams became screwed up as well, and that something overwhelmingly embarrassing happened to him! Thankfully these were only the irrational yearnings of deep sleep.

But it *was* difficult to link the walking exercises with looking up, keeping my legs wider apart, as clever as I thought I was, until I suddenly remembered in a flash that J.J. Stewart, the great New Zealand rugby coach, who became a friend during the World Rugby Seminar in the early 1980s in Cardiff, had once told me a true story, when he agreed to come over to coach Leinster for a session, during the time that I was their coach. 'Bruce Robertston,' he said, 'one of our star centre threequarters, played for a year or so in France and learned that the old accepted idea of taking and giving a pass, accompanied by the customary exaggerated swing of the hips, to maintain the correct passing movement, was as self-defeating as it was unnecessary. It was even counter-productive. Receiving and giving rugby passes, as they did in France, at shoulder height, with eyes looking straight ahead, allowed for quicker passing, faster ball movement, but better still, a more panoramic view of the whole pitch, the whereabouts of the supporting players and the placement of the opposing forces. Peripheral vision, that's what it was.'

That and many other tips made perfect sense and were adopted with alacrity by the Leinster players, who were highly impressed by 'J.J.'s' practicalities and philosophy. It was tremendous, just a few years later, to watch the Australian touring team, who played in Ireland in the mid-1980s, on their Four Countries Tour, move the ball so rapidly from one player to the next as they scanned the whole playing arena. This form of passing has been adopted universally ever since, most certainly by Ireland from 1984 onwards, when I was Irish coach.

Looking upwards, fixing my gaze on the haughty-looking clock on the end-wall, became part of the routine; it was now easier for me to remember to look up, keeping my feet apart, and with all the other things I had to do, it seemed like second nature and made far more sense. If I had been asked to stick a sweeping brush up my rear-end and sweep up the floor behind me, as I shuffled along, it would not have seemed as illogical then as it does now.

The experience resembled making the usual common mistakes while learning to water-ski: pull on the rope too hard and you're liable to fall on your bum; hold it too loosely and you could pitch on your face. Getting your legs right, your angle of lying back in the water comfortable, the towrope correctly placed and letting the boat itself pull you upright always worked for me – eventually. But not before I had collided with a shoal or two of flying fish in Barbados years before during my maiden voyage.

I often almost wept when I thought of the sprint-training I did with Edinburgh Wanderers in 1966–67 on the back pitch at Murrayfield; and all the extra private stuff outside the ground proper, on the tarmacadam walks, during the international rugby season and prior to Ireland's tour to Australia in 1967.

Being the only 'open' club in Edinburgh in the late 1960s, it was home to many misfits like me – Ronnie Lamb our Captain, John Douglas of Scotland, Lions and racehorse fame, Davy Whyte, Bill Crowe, Phil Carter, David Anderson, Terry Ellsmere and a host of other brilliant mates.

I loved it there; with UCD in Dublin it was the most enjoyable rugby ever. I was newly married to Lynne then, living in Belford Place; study and work was enjoyable at MAFF Lasswade, the rugby was brilliant and I had nothing to worry about. Strokes were of another world.

After one murder of a game against Glasgow High School FP, we all dragged ourselves off the pitch hanging on to each other for support. I overheard one craggy wing-forward say to his mountainous companion 'You know, Ewan, I *heard* some bloke kick my head in the third last ruck.' It was then I really knew what we Edinburgh 'townies' were up against!

Anyway, I tried to keep my focus on the distant clock, but with the said timepiece advancing, receding and changing position maddeningly, like a log floating in the sea, it became increasingly difficult to see things clearly. All the peripheral distractions of the other patients indulging busily in their own exercise regimes added to my difficulty in concentrating on that infuriating clock. I obviously wasn't single-minded enough yet.

Now, more than ever, it struck me that I hadn't worn spectacles for a few months, since 14 July to be exact, and I needed them badly. I couldn't see straight.

That was the next major hurdle, but a much easier one.

It had become patently obvious by now that I was in need of real assistance with my eyesight and certainly felt at a distinct disadvantage in the gym. I was therefore glad to be able to see the cursed clock a bit better after my visit to ophthalmic guru Dr Michael Browne at the Blackrock Clinic. I knew Mick well: we

ZERO POINT ONE SIX

had played rugby and tennis together, gone on holidays and generally socialised a lot. We had also left plenty of sweat on training grounds, especially Stradbrook during the mid-1970s with Blackrock College Rugby Club.

It was terribly awkward for me to be confined to a lowly wheelchair now while Mick pushed me from the car to the clinic, up to his rooms and back down to the car. I was happy though that such an old friend had helped Mandy and myself, but it did feel ridiculous to be so dependent.

The first pair of specs since my brain haemorrhage were fairly thick, with opaque edges to keep my dubious sight focused straight ahead, to suit the gym work. Peripheral vision was nearly impossible with these goggles; if I wished to see something off to the side I had to turn my head and look at it head-on.

Still, I was getting there. The formerly frustrating clock was rapidly becoming a familiar landmark. The new specs did a lot to coax my attitude and confidence along; I felt like a kid with a new suit, a poser in a playground.

No one can make you feel inferior without your consent.
(Eleanor Roosevelt, *Catholic Digest*, 1960)

It was rather striking to see the quietly determined air of industry surrounding incapacitated residents, almost like a halo; if not, then certainly a badge of membership, and I was impressed, almost to inspiration, by the unassuming professionalism of all the physios. They helped in a huge way to facilitate our transformation into recovering humans, often forcefully orchestrating this mountainous shift, and gently persuading our rehabilitation efforts by their very attitudes, since we were all encouraged to leave aside any remnants of immaterial baggage that may have accumulated, like unwanted human hair, during our previous existence.

Just like the stripping away of successive layers of onions, life there was reduced to its simplest construction, brought down to the I-want-to-get-better status, where the overwhelming majority of us merely wanted to get on with the business of adapting to our new-found circumstances. We behaved like freshly arrived tourists, getting to know their way around a new holiday resort. We were all desperate to pick up the suddenly unravelled threads and patterns of our former lives, particularly those of us who hadn't been altered in any major way by a stroke for example, and enter the so-called civilised world again as soon as it was practicable. We had been forced to become entirely new people, even though, for some, this had taken time to register.

Incredibly, some people didn't appear to be overly burdened by their enforced infirmities, accepting them as blips, albeit serious ones, on life's radar screen; they regarded the Rehab Hospital as a sort of purgatory, where they were prepared to accept for an indeterminate period all the embarrassments and setbacks that the place seemed to regard as 'normality'. I admired their faith as they knuckled down to the difficult journey back to becoming whole again. Time passed painfully slowly for us all.

Some people would certainly get there, but most would have to wait a little while longer for the anticipated recovery, and even quite a few would make relatively good progress, despite being left with a lingering imperfection of some sort.

But still there were others, fortunately the very few, who amazingly did not make the necessary efforts to help the physios look after them properly, for they apparently did not seem to care what might happen to them; or maybe they just simply lay down in the face of the tragedy that had befallen them. Instead of putting up a fierce resistance, they appeared too overcome by everything and settled for the less painful but more roundabout route back to some normality. Thankfully, they were in a tiny minority. It appeared that absolutely everything that had occurred had been part of a nasty conspiracy to thwart these people. They didn't seem to know how or where to begin to fight back against life's inequalities. They looked lost, as if they had arrived in the middle of a screen performance.

But the aura of sadness and acquiescence that enveloped them mainly prompted instant commiseration, even pity, especially towards their unfortunate relatives for being at their wits' end, not knowing how to motivate them. We were amazed that somebody would not rebel, for these less fortunate patients were surely in critical need of well-directed, professional, psychological assistance; it might have been the kind of spark they needed to give them the necessary crank-start. It was as if it would take a shock to shake them out of their lethargic sleep. Long before they ever made it through the portals of the National Rehabilitation Hospital, they should have received some form of counselling.

I knew that I could not afford to be associated with anything, or anybody negative, so I kept to myself.

Over the following weeks I came to admire the calm manner in which some patients took to their new arms, hands or legs, amazing us all with their seeming ready acceptance; they worked away doggedly, trying to become accustomed to these new gadgets. Their gritty facial expressions testified to the fact that, after the initial strivings of learners, they quickly sensed success with all their rehabilitation efforts, as doubt and uncertainty gave way to the increasing confidence of familiarity; these patients showed the rest of us that they were overcoming their unfortunate handicaps. It was a new world for me: a silent motivation movie. One could almost picture them envisaging themselves with a new limb!

We were often frozen in our tracks, held in suspended animation, as we took time out from our own toils to observe the progress of others. It was a lesson in self-preservation, in the resilience of the human spirit and in the depth of the hitherto uncharted wells of determination. We were all delighted at their success; their perseverance acted as a match to ignite the fire of our renewed resolve.

For example, I saw a woman being fitted with an artificial leg, at just about mid-thigh level, during my early days in the gym. She had maintained her sense of humour and extrovert personality throughout, earning huge respect at the no-nonsense way she became accustomed to her new limb; she had to work extremely hard to master the unfamiliar techniques. We all admired her enormously, revelled in her success, and privately we thanked her for her fortitude and example. We felt in unison with her. I never got the chance to tell her, but she had an incredibly positive effect on me.

I kept repeating to myself prayer-like 'Where there's life, there's hope.' Like most people, I had often blandly accepted those sentiments but it was all mere lip-service compared to the reality of the present. It served as a timely reminder, though, of human frailties and of the resolve to recover.

Suddenly mundane tasks like walking or moving one's fingers assumed enormous proportions, posing almost insurmountable obstacles, like the twenty-mile 'wall' in a marathon. This mental barricade can stop the uninitiated from continuing any further than twenty or so miles, so that they end up walking to finish the race.

I found that life was a constant tug-of-war between leaving behind the despondencies and shock of my afflictions, and taking on the newer, recharged feelings of the acceptance, optimism and hope for the different life that lay ahead; those twin-terrors, optimism and hope, always seemed to be at each other's throats, always in conflict, like quarrelsome in-laws.

However, there is no doubt that 'old Nick' is forever on the look-out for weakness; the dressing-gown woven of positiveness and expectation in which you wrap yourself always has many devils whispering in your ear as well, trying to sidetrack you into

settling for the easy route; these sweet nothings often develop into a roar, as you continue to make steady progress against all the odds. There is no easy route, believe me; no short cuts and little room for armchair athletics.

Success to us was relative but became the raison d'être of our existence, even when measured only in seemingly minor achievements. Optimism often finds itself shipwrecked in the sea of negativity which can accompany you into hospital; sometimes it can seem like superfluous luggage which is being constantly battered by the storms of uncertainty.

Your mental *identikit* from a previous existence will find a mirror-image in hospital, and that is why the services of trained psychologists are such a vital component of recovery. It should never be left to the patients to ask for help. It should be obligatory, like gym work.

Looking objectively at us, as we strove to go about our various tasks with singular intent, gave one the distinct feeling that while we had been provided with rough keys to our new lives, we were expected to grind them down properly ourselves into the smoother shapes that would fit better into the personal locks controlling all our destinies.

It is often remarked that behind every great man is a great woman (I'd love to meet the patronising wimp who first said that!), but certainly behind every invalid is an incredible family and an indomitable spirit, which even the floodwaters of failure cannot overwhelm.

The Rehabilitation Hospital epitomised for me the constant struggle for good to emerge victorious; negativism would have died of starvation there and hurry was a word on the prohibited list. You left impatience behind you at the entrance, like a pair of shoes when entering a Japanese tea-house.

Even though the Rehab Hospital was situated mentally on the outskirts of civilisation and on the far shores of normal living, I found that I had to create my own Berlin Wall, my own shell, while I was in there, to keep me safe from anything that could threaten me in my vulnerable state. This safety cocoon incorporated most protective mechanisms that I could muster and included a few mental long jumps as well that kept me at a distance from anything which might adversely affect me. I couldn't jump very far from a wheelchair anyway, but my wheels kept me safe!

Life had stealthily taken on a new purpose, a slow-motion urgency that was utterly compelling, far sharper and less disjointed than before; it assumed a more well-defined focus, more of an oil painting than just a pen and ink sketch. Suddenly, we were all forced to realise that the broad wish to get better was only a framework on which the new route-map, with directions on how to get there, slowly began to emerge and take shape. Living in such a close-knit community was a definite help to me and obviously I wasn't the only victim there.

The old Chinese saying that 'A journey of a thousand miles begins with a single step' had become highly relevant. Fortunately, with all the benefits of clarity and a relatively favourable prognosis, I felt like a long-distance runner being given a half-mile head-start on my comrades, in a five-mile race! I may have had a long journey stretching out in front of me, but I had a great advantage on everyone else; it made me realise just how fortunate I really was.

While I was struggling towards normality in the Rehab, I laughed out loud whenever I remembered an incident just before Ireland's first Test in Tokyo in 1985. The Japanese Prince and Princess were very much delayed in being presented to both teams, which had been lined up facing each other for about twenty extra minutes. Despite the heat and humidity the players become cold, and I was dispatched to the dressing rooms for 'hot muscle-rubs' while we all waited.

Eventually as the Princess preceded the Prince down the line of Irish players, one well-known Corkman shook her extended digits with a handful of Deep Heat. She was suitably unimpressed and said something to the Prince. He in turn very

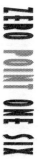

gingerly shook the player's hand, to be told by yer man, 'You're going to have trouble with yer woman tonight!' The hilarity knew no boundaries.

John Murphy's words careered monotonously around my head: 'Remember, Mick, you're just starting out at the point that most people desperately want to reach.' How true.

With my aspirations firmly anchored nearer the ground, retrieved from the imaginary land of the fairies, I concentrated on the first faltering steps that I had to master before I could begin to walk again, leaving any further thoughts of progress to dreams. In here I had ceased to be Mick Doyle the veterinarian, or the company director, the journalist, or the coach, or whatever. Instead, I had become a complete unknown – beloved of singer Bob Dylan, but certainly not a rolling stone; most certainly I was gathering moss, and like everyone else I needed help and guidance.

Pity was precious little use to me now, and, thankfully, I never experienced any of it either, by word, deed or body language. What I did need, though, were wheelbarrows full of motivation; pity wouldn't get this baby washed. I got help in abundance and trusted the staff completely. I knew I was in the right place for getting better.

Mick pointed mischievously down at his running shoes, all battered and out of shape, exclaiming, 'Sonia O'Sullivan's refused to wear these runners, I'll have you know.'

Cousin Liam and I took an amused look at these unsafe-looking specimens and retorted, 'We don't blame her; we wouldn't be seen dead in them either!'

Mick was from the Midlands and with his smiling face and

perpetually bright disposition he was a great tonic to meet and chat to on the way to the gym.

Along the wall forming part of the enclosed corridor surrounding the central garden was a set of parallel bars for walking, as in the gymnasium. Mick was learning to walk again, like many of us, but he repeated his efforts on his own, on this private Silverstone racetrack; his progress was improving too and he kept us all in good humour with his brightness and banter. He often worked at his walking in the gym in the afternoons, when it was less crowded.

If ever any unwelcome ghosts were tagging along with you on your way to the physios, you would almost be compelled to leave them with Mick; he made them disperse like swimmers in the sea who suddenly catch sight of a shark. He was a constant landmark during all the time I was in the Rehab Hospital – and never complained about anything. And I'm sure he could have. I never learned his second name, but if he happens to read this, I would like him to know that I wish him well and that I will never forget the motivation his bubbly attitude gave me always.

I gradually fell into my own regular routines of self-improvement with John Murphy in the gym. The work was just more of the same: exercise-bed, leg-weight warm-ups, stomach-muscle contraction exercises (to help my eventual walking), limited calisthenics or exercise-ball 'games' on the central mats, the walking routine on the walkways, the 'Grand Old Duke of York' extravaganzas on the steps, and pedalling to pre-set procedures on the exercise bike. While the complete programme was tremendous, and I was making definite leaps, I was utterly whacked at the end of an hour and a quarter. I often dreaded the second session in the afternoons.

They tried me once in Occupational Therapy but I was a bit

too advanced for it and not the ideal candidate for their routine games and tasks.

I tried the next-door games room later, where my balance (as I stayed within reach of my wheel-locked wheelchair) was further tested. The co-ordination between hands, legs and eyes was a bit of a lottery and while throwing heavy balls at an object, like in pitch and toss, was within my relative capabilities, I found that my attempts at table tennis were worse than any beginner's, no matter how many eyes I closed. I had all the actions and strokes off pat and would have given a table-tennis specialist a run for his or her money on any promotion video, but I couldn't hit the elusive ball, not even once. Liam told me, as diplomatically as he could, that I didn't even come near it. So much for technique and diplomacy; I gave it up as a bad job. Obviously I had oodles of ping but very little pong!

In the summer evenings of late September (I had spent about four weeks in the Rehab) I often went for drives with Mandy and Emma, down to Bray, Greystones and Brittas Bay. The Sugarloaf, Blainroe Golf Club and McDaniel's pub in Brittas became familiar, welcome landmarks. Exactly twelve years earlier Mandy and I had had our first date there – a drink in McDaniel's. It was the start of a new life for me, and I was rapidly falling in love with her – I was officially separated, I had a flourishing veterinary consultancy practice and pharmaceutical business, and had just been appointed Ireland's rugby coach. I was young (forty-four), fit and free, Mandy was twenty-seven, and Emma was just a lascivious thought. Life seemed full then.

What a change a brain haemorrhage made to everything! We were now having to start all over again.

Andrew took me on these regular trips on alternate evenings. In his late twenties he was an excellent rugby player and a good

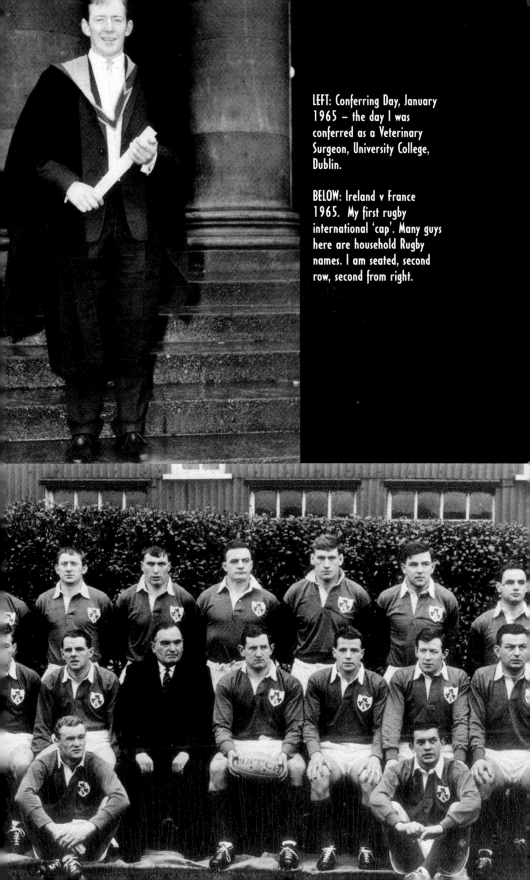

LEFT: Conferring Day, January 1965 – the day I was conferred as a Veterinary Surgeon, University College, Dublin.

BELOW: Ireland v France 1965. My first rugby international 'cap'. Many guys here are household Rugby names. I am seated, second row, second from right.

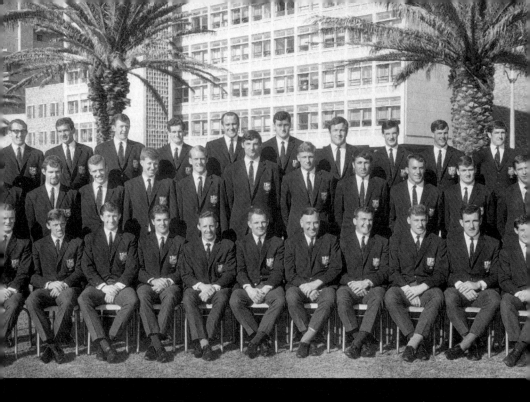

ABOVE: June 1968. British and Irish Lions tour to South Africa. Team photograph in front of Cape Town's Eden Roc Hotel. Third from left, back row, minus moustache — that's me!

BELOW: November 1998 – 30th reunion. Thirty years a growing — less (grey) hair and more weight! Dalmahoy Hotel, Edinburgh, Scotland. The fat one, second from left, plus moustache — that's me!

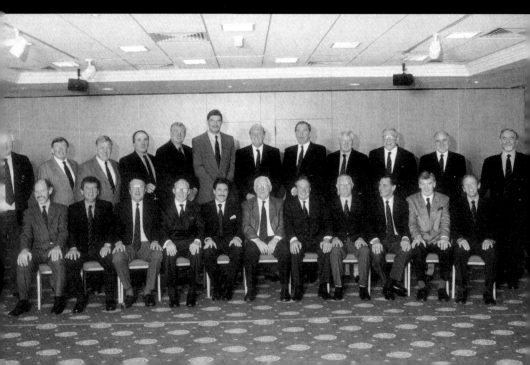

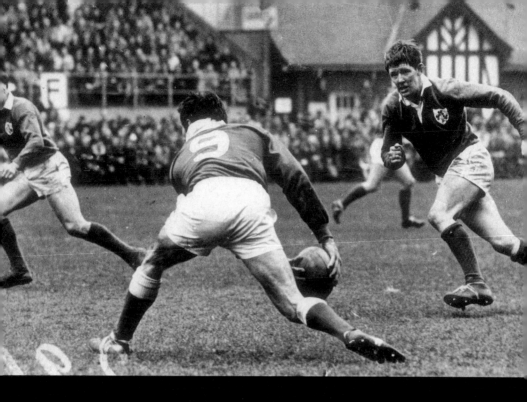

ABOVE: Ireland v Wales 1968
Brother Tom (right) and I keeping a watching brief on Gareth Edwards.

BELOW: June 1974. Dan McCarthy (left) – President Blackrock College RFC,
Fergus Slattery and myself, Captain for 1974–75.

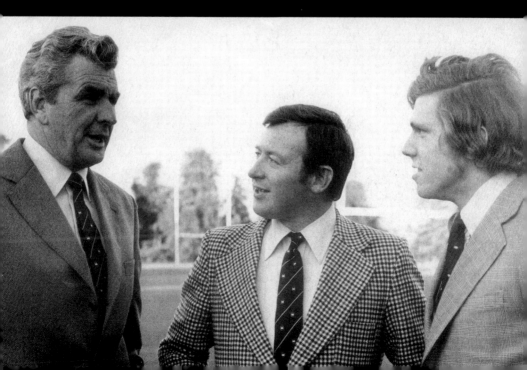

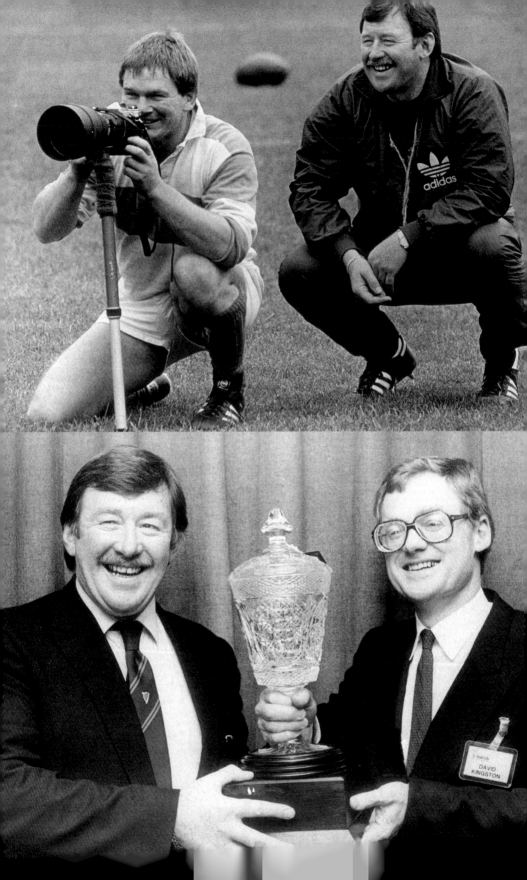

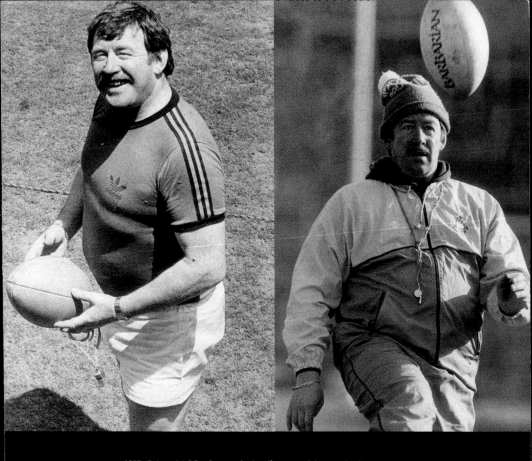

LEFT: Tokyo 1985. During Ireland's tour of Japan, looking carefree at a training session before the first Test.

RIGHT: Dublin 1986. Squad training before Ireland v Scotland. The proceedings obviously didn't warrant my input!

OPPOSITE PAGE:
ABOVE: February 1985. Irish Rugby Captain Ciaran Fitzgerald and myself at a squad coaching session, Landsdowne Road, Dublin.

BELOW: April 1985. David Kingston, Chief Executive Irish Life, presenting me with the Manager of the Year Award. I haven't dropped it yet.

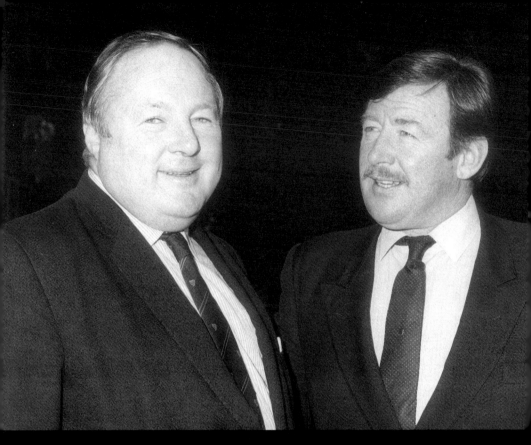

ABOVE: Circa 1985, Dublin. Michael Cuddy, Chairman of Selectors for Leinster and then Ireland – later President of the I.R.F.U. – and me.

BELOW: August 1985. McCarthy's Pub, Fethard, Co. Tipperary. During a memorable weekend with the Irish Team at Coolmore Stud. I was pulling pints of Guinness for Irish team members (left to right) Philip Orr, myself, Donal Lenihan and Willie Anderson.

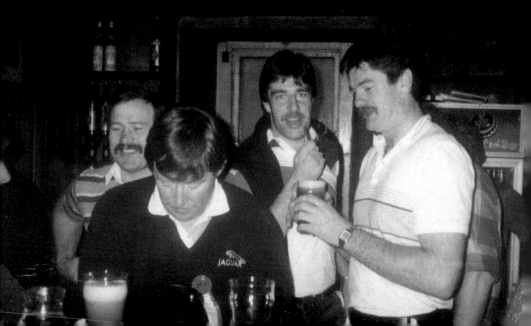

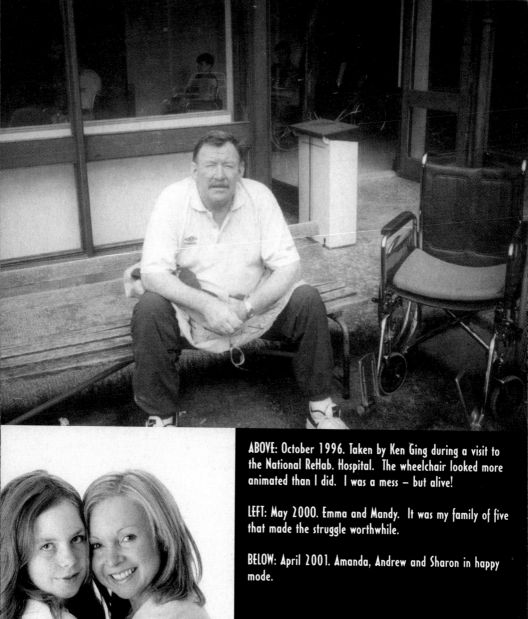

ABOVE: October 1996. Taken by Ken Ging during a visit to the National ReHab. Hospital. The wheelchair looked more animated than I did. I was a mess – but alive!

LEFT: May 2000. Emma and Mandy. It was my family of five that made the struggle worthwhile.

BELOW: April 2001. Amanda, Andrew and Sharon in happy mode.

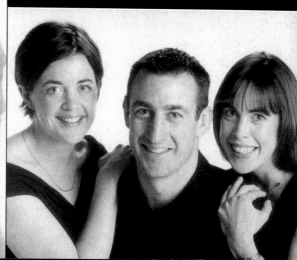

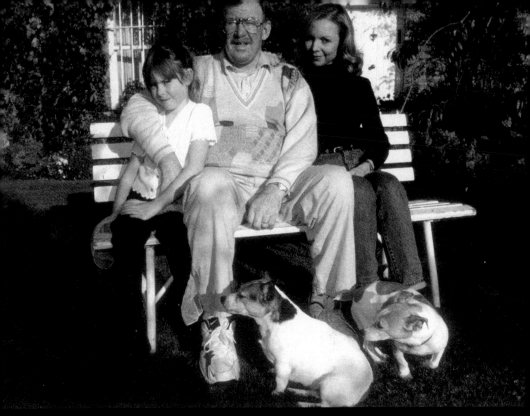

ABOVE: Mandy, Emma and myself with 'friends' Buntie and Tiffin in front of home;
I had just left the ReHab. hospital for the last time and look suitably confused.

BELOW: May 2001. Photo of Daisy ('Nurse Nancy') and myself trying
to look intelligent for the camera. I failed!

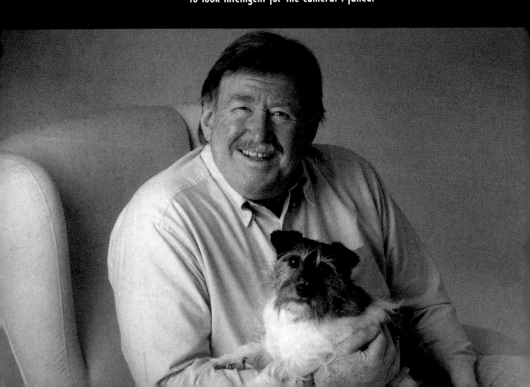

bloke – a great friend to me. I was naturally proud of his football achievements at school in Blackrock College and afterwards with Landsdown Rugby Club. His marketing position with Mars/Master Foods suited his talents admirably and I just loved going off on motor trips with him; I felt safe with him driving. We usually came home by Jack White's pub on the main Arklow–Dublin road; of course, Jack White's has achieved front-page notoriety with all the revelations during the trial and conviction of co-owner Catherine Nevin for the murder of her husband Tom, the other proprietor. Innocent then, it has attracted unwelcome fame for different reasons since.

I loved being out in the open, revelling in the change of scenery from hospital, the superb views and the freedom. I looked forward to, indeed depended incredibly, on these jaunts, and then miraculously found my room filling up with visitors when I arrived back at the hospital. They were like exhausted birds nesting in the evenings after a day's busy toil.

I'm sure that the uninitiated were mildly surprised not to find a jabbering wreck confined to a bed of pain, but nevertheless we were all delighted to meet again. I won't bother you with their names, but I *was* always glad to see them all. An odd visitor's presence escapes my memory now, and this infrequent lapse has since made me feel a fool at times.

Hospitals are amazing places; while I was obviously too ill in Beaumont to appreciate apples and oranges, I was given lots of fruit and chocolate in the Rehab. The ubiquitous grapes figured large in my fruit bowl. Now you'd think that the fruit was mainly for the patients and probably a relative to have the odd munch; however, some visitors felt that the grapes were designated for them alone, in appreciation of their presence, and would scoff the bloody lot unless you told them to buzz off and buy their own. The Grapes of Wrath syndrome.

It *was* good to have all my old friends visit me in hospital; these were rugby pals mostly. Their visits and chats spurred me on, guaranteeing my resolve to meet them all again on the outside, as equals; if not to take up exactly where we had left off, then to get as close as possible to it.

One of my regular visitors in the Rehab was Michael Cuddy; he had been Chairman of the Leinster and Ireland selectors when I was coach. We had always enjoyed a tremendously successful fun time together. His wife Meda and two young daughters were killed in a car/truck accident in the late 1980s, leaving Michael and his only son John grief-stricken.

However, he weathered the storm bravely. He later met our friend Helen Buckley, whom he married. The night before their wedding, as Leinster finished a training session at Donnybrook, Eddie Thornton (last year's Leinster president) presented him with a set of jump leads, with the pointed advice, 'Never arrive at home sober, Cud, or the wife'll know for sure that you take a drink!' Great memories, especially when you are invalided in bed.

I fell into the normal routine of being woken at about eight o'clock by the nurse, as she recorded my temperature and blood pressure and helped me to take my tablets. I shaved, washed and got dressed while I hovered not too far from my wheelchair, taking the lift down to the breakfast room to join the queues of Hungry Harrys.

After breakfast, which entailed meeting and eating with different people, all the while helping to expand my circle of friends, I sauntered off on my wheels, usually to talk to Mick on the way to the gym. A morning session in the Palace of Gain was followed by another in the afternoon, separated by lunch. The food was reasonably good; I was amazed that a menu was displayed on a blackboard in the corridor every day. I had lost my taste for everything but chicken, sausages, eggs, bread and jam, and tea. Any food such as beef or lamb left a queer taste and I couldn't eat it – anything fatty had become distasteful all of a sudden.

In between times I lay on my bed and listened to the radio. I rediscovered RTE Radio 1, listening avidly to the news and

ZERO POINT ONE SIX

other programmes of interest. My eldest daughter Sharon had brought me a CD/radio and discs in Beaumont Hospital, to help my progress, but I could now listen to them much better in the Rehab – Ruth Rendell mysteries receiving a lot of air-time.

There was a regular pattern to my life now. A normal person would probably become bored with such tedium, but I was delighted. Still I craved going home soon and dreaded my legs becoming itchy every night just when I should be going to sleep.

'He was born an Englishman and remained one for years.'
(Brendan Behan, *The Hostage*, 1958)

One morning on my way to lectures at the Veterinary College in Ballsbridge I came across Brendan Behan, author, poet, playwright and unique celebrity, probably feeling the effects of the night before, dressed in a fur coat and hailing an 'effing taxi'; the effing taxi came in effing quick time, Brendan piled in and effed off. I never actually met him but admired him enormously. Some of his observations and writings were brilliant and I do regret, like most, that the drink eventually got to him.

He once claimed that he was 'a drinker with a writing problem', but boozing and bravura camouflaged his real worth. His *Borstal Boy*, *The Hostage* and *The Quare Fella* are still classics. Sadly, he passed away too early, having done much too little. The above quote from *The Hostage*, though, does remind me acutely of something I developed latterly while in Beaumont and of another, altogether different, affliction, that had even predated the brain haemorrhage: during Easter Week 1995 it was postulated that I might have a slight kidney infection and the appropriate preventative antibiotics were prescribed. I rapidly developed a numbness in the first three fingers of my right hand, the right half of both lips and the right side of my face.

This numbness was present in my fingers and lips when the

subarachnoid haemorrhage hit me, but when I woke up a few weeks later, there was full feeling miraculously in those previously affected zones. However, after a while the numbness returned and still persists in all its glory, waiting, I suppose, to die with me. To make it even worse I didn't have *any* kidney infection after all!

Then one evening, weeks after I woke up in Beaumont, I felt an unusual sensation in my feet, particularly my right one. They were hot and sore and twitched involuntarily. Mandy and I called them 'wayward legs' and only sleeping tablets would allow me to get past the first two hours of extreme discomfort. I tried nearly everything except amputation.

The Beaumont staff were able to keep the twitching under control, but in the Rehab Hospital they seemed reluctant to give me the much sought-after, extremely mild Normesin sleeping tablets. So, the wayward legs continued, even getting progressively worse, and I'm sure that many visitors wondered what all the movement was about under the bedclothes around nine o'clock at night! It wasn't me, yer Lordship.

The condition stayed with me during my stay in the Rehab Hospital; I had to keep on begging for those blasted sleep-inducing pills to help me get over the constant nightly irritation. I believed that daytime activity kept the soreness and twitching at bay, but as soon as I was lying on my back in bed, after a few hours of quiet every evening, the condition began with an almost alarm-clock-like regularity.

Professor Eóin O'Brien confirmed that the very condition, actually termed 'wayward legs', had been written up in the *Sunday Times* supplement about a decade or so earlier and that either librium, valium, uranium or strontium had been prescribed! The danger, of course, was that some of these tablets might be habit-forming and could lead to addiction or some form of dependence.

I reckoned that pressure on the nerves around my lower back and bottom contributed to the numbness that accompanied my wayward legs, and that the multiple activities of later on would lead to an end to the discomfort. Anyway, a few months after going home, about November 1996, I finally got rid of this affliction, and luckily it has only intermittently made its appearance since.

Unlike Brendan Behan's Englishman, it remained with me only for some time, like a bad cold; but I am now glad to miss it. One of the few examples of activity that I was happy to get rid of.

SEVEN

Dreams from a Wheelchair

Motivation assumes many guises, expressing itself in different ways. Basically, I wanted to get past the wheelchair phase and leave the Rehab Hospital as whole and as fast as I could.

During the first few weeks there, life was like a runaway train, with its own head of steam; I almost just sat on for the ride. I was delighted to be swept along on a tide of 'can doisms' and could hardly help getting on to the right track. The atmosphere and philosophy of the place stimulated hitherto dormant determination to wake up and go about things properly. I found the positiveness infectious; we were all in the same boat, all there to get well. We all had one-track minds: just to improve and go home.

While Beaumont had represented survival: life or death, the Rehab painted a broader outline of a new life, coaxing me to put a brain and a heart into the bony skeleton, to become myself again. The everyday things – exercising, eating, setting off on drives, meeting family and friends – signalled that a more normal life was gradually returning.

Every new achievement of my fellow-patients, even a couple of extra steps, a few balancing exercises more, was felt by all of us and recorded as a significant gain. I knew that I could not let

ZERO POINT ONE SIX

myself remain physically or mentally incapacitated. I felt that if I could stand, I could walk; if I could walk, I could drive and I could think – and I could become normal.

As the coach to intelligent, gifted players I had always followed a private dictum, no matter what our goals happened to be, of 'realistic expectations with tolerance of imperfections'. Our players were an amalgam of careers, professions and intelligence levels (they were all, repeat all, very clever), politics and religions. Whenever they put on the jerseys of their province or of Ireland, their private lives became public, even for a short while, and their rugby philosophies coalesced into *performance* and *success*.

On rugby teams, career roles are quite often reversed: a bloke on a team may, as its captain or pack leader, be in charge of someone who is his actual boss in their daily working life; rugby, like brain haemorrhage, is a great leveller.

It is often said that a career based on status, financial security and simple economics is a difficult one if you're a nurse; a vocation is reckoned to be more essential, or more desirable. I have no doubt whatever now that money alone could not compensate the staff in the Rehab Hospital. They needed to have been deeply dedicated to make this their profession. I found that their patience, their caring, their almost resigned drive, encouragement and laid-back coolness were major factors in my improvement.

They couldn't *act* like that all the time; it had to have been a 'calling'. There is little doubt now that they were always 'tolerant of my imperfections'. I owe them such a lot; my life in fact.

'All' I had to do with this runaway racehorse was to hold on, guaranteeing that my own physical attributes (gaining in strength and value by the day), and my awakening motivation kept pace. Together we could do it; alone, we were doomed. Interdependent.

The trust, the expectation of self-help that the staff had of the patients in the Rehab Hospital, rubbed off on all of us, adding significant values to our hymn books of achievement. Realistic expectations . . .

If I appear to be eulogising the Rehab Hospital at the expense of Beaumont, I don't mean to do so in any way at all; what I'm trying to do is to emphasise that while the medical side of things took precedence over everything else in Beaumont, in the Rehab, rehabilitation and repair dwarfed all else. They were two totally different institutions, with separate agendas that distinguish them, but both were vital to people like me. Without the emergency surgery, the Intensive and Coronary Care and the attention to detail that always existed for me in Beaumont, then the Rehab Hospital, no matter how central to my return journey, would not have mattered for me.

This of course does not imply that both are holiday camps, that their patients have a free ride, and that both are so perfect that improvements cannot be made. That would be incorrect. Both hospitals should exist of course for the primary benefit of patients; and patient care must always come first. I've often wondered if it actually does! I hope so.

Being encouraged to entertain visitors, to head off on drives or out to restaurants, going home from Friday to Sunday nights and all the little normal things, these signified that life was becoming more normal, and that I could be entrusted to the care of my own family without being too much of a burden on them; even though I now know that I was then an extremely awkward sod.

Obviously I was making the necessary progress with John Murphy, but I was ready for a new challenge.

She arrived out of the blue, one Monday morning and she meant business. *She* was Ann Keane and she became my other physio. Just as fingerprints can vary between people, Ann brought a different variation to the same theme. While there aren't many

different ways of putting one foot in front of the other, there *are* changes of emphasis on how to go about it.

I soon learned that it was hospital policy for physios to alternate between patients, to simply act as a new stimulus. While part of me regretted the loss of John, who had by now become an old friend, I was delighted to have Ann as my new helper, together with the fresh challenges she represented. The male/female relationship possibly prompted me to be on my best behaviour too.

We basically did more of the same, but a few variations became obvious fairly quickly. She decided one morning that I was going to walk the length of the gym – no arguments. I did too, much to the surprise of myself and the amazement of most onlookers. I began to look forward to more and more walking, always supported by Ann holding my arm. It helped me make the breakthrough.

It felt as if I had broken the four-minute-mile barrier alongside Roger Bannister, the first sub-four-minute miler back in those distant 1950s days at Oxford University. That 150 feet of gym-length was quite a milestone and represented real recovery. I had stumbled over an almost impossible hurdle and it felt great. The Phoenician warriors had nothing on me – as they went into battle *they* had only been exhorted to 'Come back with your shields or on them!', whereas I had to escape the physical and mental ruts that my vivid imagination had created, and which were now holding me back.

Ann rapidly introduced kicking a football to me, to stretch my powers of balance and reaction time to the absolute limit; I had to make constant adjustments to my eternally taxed co-ordination. But at least I could see the ball this time, not like the table-tennis episode when I often belted fresh air into subjugation!

Normally, women are not as adept at ball-kicking as men, but Ann was in the ascendancy. Gradually, I improved at the gym-walking and the kicking skills and both of us got a little bolder,

ZERO POINT ONE SIX

venturing to walk out on to the quadrangle around the central flowerbeds. Unfortunately, the transition from the natural brightness of the gym to the lower intensity lighting of the corridor bamboozled me, causing a serious hindrance to my walking ability. This continues to a lesser extent today. So we gave it up as a bad idea; but this was only a minor hiccough. It merely represented an exercise that was beyond me – for the moment.

Ann came from Skerries, a north County Dublin seaside town, and was well accustomed to rugby types. Skerries was home to many of my friends – Bill and Christine Mulcahy and Jim and Helen Glennon among them. I knew Ann's aunt, Patricia, well and our families had (mis)spent many a raucous Sunday in the early seventies, in the company of her uncle-in-law, Phelim, in her folks' Bus Bar.

Ann's familiarity with all things oval allowed her to say with conviction, 'You're a typical rugby type, Mick: you have a concentration span of about ninety minutes, during which you'll break your neck with effort, but after that, zero. And then you're ready to begin all over again after lunch!' She was right, but I couldn't help it.

Years earlier, during my early coaching days with Leinster, the players always asked me at the start of each training session, 'How long, Mick?' – ninety minutes being the limit of their attention span, too. But then they won almost every game anyway over our five years from 1979 to 1984! They were right.

Eventually Ann took up a job in a hospital nearer home and I found myself back in the capable hands of Maestro Murphy. Though very different, they were both superb helpers.

My mental state was catching up fast with my physical abilities; the progress I was making in the gym and elsewhere, although not earth-shattering to normal civilians, was astounding in my case. Things were beginning to work in synchrony at last. That was a huge psychological uplift, capable of wafting me along effortlessly on its tide.

I thoroughly enjoyed my sole swim in the pool, entertained about sixteen friends in my room on a Thursday evening and the next afternoon Mandy drove me home for the weekend. We had lunch with George and Olivia James on the way home, delighted that a feeling of normality was creeping in, to become, if not an everyday occurence, then part of my life at that time.

EIGHT

Home Sweet Home . . .

Suddenly, being at home, removed at one fell swoop from all the friendly familiar faces and the unhurried tranquillity of hospital, was a mixed blessing. The monotony, if you could ever call it that, and the necessarily orchestrated regimentation of the Rehab Hospital were telling me clearly that I was ready for the next hurdle on my recovery track, at home in Sherlockstown, County Kildare.

That and the fact that so many callers were putting a huge strain on my progress prodded me into leaving. Even welcome visitors can become a serious problem when you're struggling to get better! I certainly could not put a sign on my door saying 'Push off, family only' to all my friends, so I stayed home; in the end everything carries its own price tag – unfortunately.

The idea of finding myself at home in comfortable security with my family had enormous appeal, but I also felt an acute sense of loss for the place which had been home to me for five or six weeks: it had taken me in initially as a chair-bound invalid, and had transformed me into a human being once more: a person who was ready, though frightened and apprehensive, to begin walking in earnest again, out in the fresh air, among familiar routes and under God's sky.

At home, in the early stages, my mind was in turmoil and filled with doubt, as I wondered 'Am I doing the right thing? Will I keep missing Liam or Brendan, Marie, Kay or Mick and the others? Can I make the right level of progress without professionals like John Murphy and Ann Keane helping me?' and so on.

Against all that, everybody was glad to have me at home; it meant that I had survived the crisis and, with luck, would get much better. The regular nearness of Mandy and Emma, and Andrew, Sharon and Amanda and that of my close friends and colleagues supported me enormously at a time when I was full of self-doubt; they helped me profoundly, all willing me to make a good recovery. I couldn't let everybody down.

I looked reasonable, I suppose, for a bloke who had nearly copped it. Alive's better than dead any day, but looks can camouflage how you really feel inside; I often looked great, but felt terrible. I vividly recalled what a nurse told me as I was leaving Beaumont: 'Just remember two things, Mick: don't be in any hurry to do anything, don't forget that you have all the time you need; and second, you are competing against nobody but yourself.' She couldn't have given me a better present. Those were the principles that guided me as I replayed her exact words, so often, during all my endeavours to get better. I owe her much more than my sanity.

When I first came home I could speak reasonably well, apart from skipping odd words here and there and having trouble with recalling some names and happenings. Whereas before, when I'd mentally stumble and say 'you know, what's his name' or 'what do you call that place?', I was merely being lazy. Now I meant it!

And the Zimmer frame helped me also to get around OK. It remains in the corner of my office today – a stark memory. But mentally I still had a long way to go; I felt that I was in quite a bit of a mess, and the awful inescapable tiredness that accompanies a stroke began to manifest itself, as I undertook what everyone else regarded as mundane tasks. Even thinking about various things that I had to do knackered me!

For the first week or so I did very little, just sat down in a comfortable armchair, gathering my thoughts and ambitions and watching TV. I liked the news, sport, the History channel, crocodiles and sharks and all the nasties that are better left to the screen. I became an expert on wars as I followed the exploits of Allied and German generals during the Second World War, revelling in campaigns against the Nazis and the Japanese armies. Sky TV was highly instructive, especially the Discovery and National Geographic channels.

Our dogs had become even more important to me now and seemed to understand my plight; they were obviously delighted to have me all to themselves. When I went to bed a few of them, Jack Russells all, accompanied me on to the bed, while Rommel, the huge German Shepherd, relaxed on the corner couch. I loved having them around me.

Daisy used to lick the wound left by the drainage tubes at the back of my head that was still there five months after . . . She kept up this ritual until she had helped heal it completely. We called her Nurse Nancy.

But all this early inactivity at home was like the calm that prevailed uneasily before the storm tore into everything, shaking us out of our comfortable existences. It was as if we were all waiting for the day when Mandy and Emma took me walking again.

We all knew that the armoury of exercises, the efforts and the rapid advance that I had made in Dún Laoghaire were merely preparation for actually walking outside. It was akin to learning to ride a bicycle for the first time. So here goes, I thought, in at the deep end, as I left my lifebelt behind at home.

It was exciting though, this learning to walk all over again. I had to tense my stomach muscles, as I'd been told, to make walking and balancing easier, and to keep my feet much farther apart initially, which they had also drilled into me in the Rehab Hospital.

I began improving gradually. With Emma walking backwards in front of us, Mandy on one side, holding on to me, and the security of the aluminium walking-stick on the other, I made slow but steady progress; only fifty yards or so at first and then we extended it gradually until I could walk, supported, for about a quarter of a mile at a time along the canal-bank road. It felt as if I was doing it all for the first time.

Surprisingly, I found that taking my strides relatively quickly prevented me from falling over; this inclination was a constant companion, and a fear. It became even more pronounced months later, until it progressed into a serious problem. However, for now, walking fairly rapidly became a regular feature of my navigatory efforts. Falling down sober was always a worry.

We left the dogs at home during these early walks just in case I fell over them! Besides, the road along the Grand Canal was now closed off to motorised traffic. It was quiet; we had the whole place to ourselves and because all my mistakes would be private ones, nobody else would see my infant-like first attempts.

I was reasonably sensitive about my condition initially, wondering what people might think. 'Didn't that bloke used to do something important in rugby at one time? A fit fella, he was – look at him now' kind of thing. No wonder I was self-conscious, but thankfully, pretty soon the 'I'm all right, Jack' syndrome clicked in and I really didn't give a fiddler's what anybody thought of me. Even if anybody *had* noticed, they probably wouldn't care a toss anyway.

Luckily also, the road surface, though devoid of tarmac, was reasonably smooth; otherwise I couldn't have negotiated it. I really hated any unevenness in this new, strange condition. Potholes had to be avoided.

After a few weeks I progressed from this semi-private canalway to a mile walk along the Grand Canal road up past Sallins, then to a two-mile trek farther along the canal towards the village of Prosperous, in the other direction. During all this time Mandy held on to me, just in case, and I even tried to wobble on my own for short stretches as I became more confident, or cheeky. I had by now grown accustomed to cars, bikes and pedestrians; it was a reasonably quiet road but still much busier than that first route. I felt like a pony being patiently trained to ignore the traffic.

During those early weeks of walking every day, with Mandy's help (Emma was in Hewetson School nearby), I gradually got into the swing again, even though my muscles felt weak and my feet wooden; they landed on the ground with each stride like solid planks – flat and awkward. But at least I was moving and I was out in the fresh air. I was making unbelievable progress, but I didn't feel that then. I was still anxious and apprehensive – would I ever become normal?

The longer route along the canal was tree-lined for much of its length and the branches, recently bare of leaves, looked down over everything in the misty stillness of late October. Their very presence along with the odd grey squirrel and occasional songbird testified that nature, even during the closed season, was still very much alive, and with my accompanying poor eyesight I could still see enough.

The dank, almost eerie quietness was like a slow intake of breath, a welcome pause before the westerly winds buffeted everything in their path. For the very first time I could understand how Percy Bysshe Shelley was prompted to write his immortal poem, 'The Ode to the West Wind':

> O Wild West Wind, thou breath of Autumn's being,
> Thou, from whose unseen presence the leaves dead
> Are driven like ghosts from an enchanter fleeing;
>
> Yellow, and black, and pale, and hectic red,
> Pestilence-stricken multitudes: O thou,
> Who chariotest to their dark wintry bed

The wingèd seeds, where they lie cold and low,
Each like a corpse within its grave, until
Thine azure sister of the Spring shall blow

Her clarion o'er the dreaming earth.

He was so observant. I wondered if he had had an infirmity like mine, allowing his imagination to prompt his powers of observation, transcending mundane thoughts and letting them take wing, comparing the fate of autumnal seeds to human corpses whereby singly they have been consigned to their graves, to awaken sometime later.

Leaves go through life's endless cycle of death and rebirth, while humankind, we hope, reawakens in blissful after-life as a reward for long toil on earth.

Shelley was certainly very profound. I was somewhat like that when I went into hospital, almost like a dying seed whose very existence was threatened, and after escaping eternity and an enforced stay in the safe but threatening cocoon of purgatory, I had come alive again, capable of making the strides required of me; strides being the operative word. At least I was going somewhere. I now felt like a flea in training for something or other – but a very tired, battered and banjaxed one.

NINE

Falling Down Sober

Between the idea
And the reality
Between the motion
And the act
Falls the Shadow.
(T.S. Eliot, 'The Hollow Men', 1925)

My early life of recovery occupied the twilight world for quite some time; a world where frightening shadows (differing altogether from my silhouette) flitted unfettered, and worries strutted around like thugs making themselves felt. Still, somewhere, near the edge of the mental horizon, I could see a tunnel in my mind's eye: a faint but definite point to aim for, as I stumbled through the whole jigsaw of uncertainty, which seemed as difficult as riding a mountain-bike through thick porridge.

I was OK while Mandy and Emma were with me, but how would I do on my own? There was only one way to find out. We went on holiday to Parknasilla in Kerry for a few weeks in late October, to get things back to normal after all the disruptions. We first met all the relations and friends at our cousin Marion's

wedding to Niall, but I felt queer and out of it, not being able to stand, dance or drink. I didn't smoke either, to complete my list of visible vices. My halo was weighing me down.

When you're on the dry, weddings aren't great fun, especially during the early days of your sobriety, but I felt secure with my aluminium walking-stick; it explained everything, without me having to say a word. However, despite my deficiencies, we had a brilliant time.

I remembered vividly one post-match cocktail reception during Ireland's summer tour to Japan in 1985. Current Lions' tour manager Donal Lenihan, even then an important veteran in rugby circles, asked his Japanese conversationalists, 'Do you have many elections here in Japan?'

One of the more brazen Japanese Hormone Harrys retorted, 'Ah, knickars.' That seemed to add a certain frisson to the rattle of glasses! A bit like the wedding, but there were no signs of any underwear anywhere.

I had to fully embrace my new life without booze, and this special gathering represented the first real group occasion to put my resolve to the ultimate test. My former inclinations were tempting me as I surreptitiously viewed all the bottles. Luckily I had my cousin Tom, Marion's dad, who hadn't taken a drink in years, to keep me company. So I didn't feel naked. I quenched the flames before they became fires.

The calm of Sunday was inexorably replaced by the storm of Monday morning, when the real business of recovery began on the beaches of Derrynane. This is a truly enchanting place. It is about a mile or so down off the main road, towards the sea, the drive passing through the carparks, past the outhouses and grounds of Derrynane Abbey, Daniel O'Connell's family home.

O'Connell, one of the greatest names of Irish history, was born in that house, lived there for most of his early life and was reputedly buried in the graveyard on the nearby island. The Irish state owns the whole estate now and during the holiday season it opens the house and gardens to visitors. Looking now at

O'Connell's armchair, and the girth of him, one would wonder how he ever fitted into it without a shoehorn. It is justifiably right and fitting that the public purse should be used for the upkeep of the birthplace of Ireland's champion of Catholic emancipation.

Down by the sea is a pier and an understated little harbour, open at one end to the Atlantic, its small mouth guarded by a giant tooth-like rock sticking up out of the water, like some strange, inanimate sentry. There is a beach, some sandhills and then a little island with a small quaint graveyard; the island is cut off regularly by the tide. To the left of the island three beaches stretch out for a few miles; these merge when the tide is out.

Fortunately, when we were there, the beaches were deserted, except for the seagulls, cormorants, the seals and the fish. Anyway, I could now fall around the place to my heart's content, unnoticed. And I often fell. It was a great place for making mistakes, unseen.

Mandy and Emma kickstarted me off walking, but after the first few hundred yards I felt that I could go ahead on my own, at a fair old pace. I soon left them behind, content to take their time and slowly wander along nonchalantly.

I had to walk fairly fast to keep my balance, which by now had become a serious problem; I had been often warned about it in Dún Laoghaire. Walking any slower was out of the question for me, because I was afraid that I would topple over at any second. Speed would keep me safe; my momentum would prevent me from falling down. The very act of standing around or walking slowly was disorientating and uncomfortable, as vertigo ruled everything.

Vertigo is a serious impediment to easy movement: I suffered from an intense fear of heights and of any uneven terrain in addition to my normal unsteadiness, and I'm afraid that the balance-centre of my brain had gone off on a world cruise, leaving me to cope with my ungainly stance. My early movements during those walks were decidedly awkward.

I didn't feel any particular sharp head pain along with the vertigo, but my brain felt woolly and I had become acutely aware of a constant feeling of numbness or dullness in my head. It is difficult to describe it, but I certainly knew that something nasty had happened to me. Sometimes the dullness developed into a more focused pain, centred on the back of my skull, where the bony cranium had been drilled to relieve the haemorrhage and drain the area of blood and stuff. It differed from the usual headache though, but enough to make things uneasy – like a constant reminder. I regularly took the Distalgesic tablets prescribed for me and felt considerable easing; I am not a tablet junkie but these ones certainly helped. I still take them occasionally.

However, nothing was allowed to interfere with my walking; it felt peculiar to be moving along the water's edge, where the sand was smooth and compacted and the water consistently lapped. It was an eerie feeling to be taking those initial awkward steps, being kept upright by the aluminium walking-stick, doing without Mandy and Emma's help and having to lean into the persistent off-sea breeze to keep myself from being blown over.

The seagulls seemed to mock my feeble efforts during the first few days of the week I spent there, as I struggled to master the new demands of following one step with another. At the time it felt like I was climbing the Himalayas with a gammy leg; I left my imprint on the sand a lot!

As the gulls began to recognise me from the days before, I imagined that their animated chattering, as they dipped to earth or soared skywards, was their way of crying out to each other in approval of my giant progress. I am not conversant with seagull-speak but I was convinced, as I forced myself to walk along the beach, that the birds were giving me a rousing ovation instead of their earlier standing boo. I even took pleasure in remembering that poor old Long John Silver had only one good leg.

The walk, there and back, was about three miles and it felt, every monotonous time I travelled it, like I had just completed a marathon; but I was really chuffed with myself that my efforts were being rewarded. Nothing like years before of course, when I had become super-fit from training during my days as an international rugby player, but real progress nevertheless. I fell down less and less as time went on.

Simple things though, like stepping on to and walking on a flat expanse of buried rock a full inch above ground level felt like a mountain climb! I had to force myself to do it and conquer this new and ridiculous fear of heights; 'heights' – blimey! – it was only ground level, not a steep hill.

Equally, getting up and down the fifteen or so steps on to the beach and walking along the two-plank-wide bridge across the stream leading from the carpark were major hurdles, requiring all the resolve and ingenuity that I could scrape together – and I'm normally a can-do person.

However, it was all good training. More and more obstacles were now materialising along the way, reminding me in case I forgot, 'Don't be so cocky, Mick, life is full of pitfalls and potholes.' I knew for certain then that the luxury of the helping hands at Beaumont and the Rehab Hospital had been well and truly amputated and I had been cut adrift.

The feeling of nausea that I had experienced weeks earlier, looking at the sea advance and recede on the seafront in Bray during a drive from the Rehab, had returned in all its glory; but while I might look directly, inadvertently, at the moving water that befuddled and confused me, the feelings of sickness in the pit of my stomach or the dullness in my head did not seem as pronounced as before.

I was obviously getting slightly better and was able to avoid looking directly at the water by walking parallel to the shore; it was almost like a TV programme – if you don't like it, zap it off with the remote control. It sounds so simple, but to ignore the sounds of the waves is easier said than done. There is always a fascinating compulsion, though, which draws one by invisible strings to look at, almost to stare at the sea.

When white-crested sea-horses race one another relentlessly across the wide expanse of water in a bay, the picture becomes registered like a cattle brand on one's consciousness. It seems to trigger thoughts of previous times when we were kids, and nostalgic, lucid visions of sandcastles, moats and buckets and spades run through our minds in a flash. All of this happened to me. Oh to be a child again!

One day Mandy drove us out to revisit Glanmore Lake, a few miles from Kenmare on the Beara Peninsula. It is a truly beautiful place, àit ann feinn (an outstanding place), lying among the hills and fields, with thousands of fir trees lending it the aura of an enchanted pleasure-spot in Norway or Sweden. The copious conifers seemed to be abseiling down along the rocks or acting as barricades to protect these weathered protuberances.

Glanmore Lake itself is fed by a musical stream and drained by a waterway at the other end, which then empties itself into a winding river that snakes its way to the sea. Initially, after it flows under a small wooden bridge, the stream is fast-moving like a narrow river.

We had often barbecued there along the picturesque banks of the stream that flowed into the lake; there are numerous holiday photos of us three, with the car, the barbecue and the smoke fitting in harmoniously with inquisitive, wary flies. The local fish must have experienced the odd culture shock too as their tranquillity was threatened.

I remembered with a twinge of pain in my heart the first time Mandy and I had come here and how much in love we were then, ten years earlier. Brain haemorrhages, by the way, do not eliminate one's ardour; they may throw cold water on it to dampen the glow of the fires for a while, but they certainly don't eliminate erotic thoughts. At least mine weren't dimmed. I obviously wasn't a Viagra candidate yet.

Anyway, I found that as a front-seat passenger on the drive to Glanmore Lake, the constant winding of the narrow country road had a disconcerting effect on my brain, as the focal distance of my eyesight shortened and suddenly lengthened again with every bend. For all the world I felt like a fiddler's elbow. Eventually I had to close my eyes altogether, ignoring the views from the car, hoping that the feelings of faintness and exasperation might pass off.

It was obvious that I had a fair way to go yet, but at least I was making progress. I kept my eyes shut on the return drive too. T.S. Eliot was absolutely right: 'the motion and the act' were in the shade at the moment, in subdued light.

———————————

It had been fascinating to see a limping Dustin Hoffman acting as a valet-type gopher in Jon Voight's quest to become a 'midnight cowboy' in the movie. It was tragic to watch the climax, in a silence interspersed with sniffing, as Voight cradled the just-dead Hoffman in his arms as they entered Los Angeles on a Greyhound bus. I'll never forget the many tragi-comic moments of that film. Even though I was far removed from being a midnight cowboy, the similarities with odd parts of my own life couldn't be discounted, except that I hadn't died; I *had* been give a second chance.

The isolation of walking on my own on the beach had now ended and it was time for me to face the public on the roads around our hotel in Parknasilla. Self-consciously I thought that everyone knew about my story or else were staring at me, but of course they weren't interested. It was just my imagination. I consoled myself with that thought anyway, even though a few people in the Great Southern Hotel recognised me.

Whereas on previous visits when I was a much fitter guest, I had set out from the hotel either running or walking back to Oysterbed Pier two miles away, or up the hills through the

Sillagh Woods, on this occasion I had to be content with erratic walking, since my balance and movement continued to embarrass me. Apart from the constant buzzing in my head, the walks to Oysterbed and the similar distance to Rosdohan Pier were incredibly gratifying and filled with nostalgia, as well as the wonder that I was still around. A big step.

I enjoyed those walks on the roads no end, but the journey up through the Sillagh Woods and the ranks of cultivated conifers along the way gave me similar problems to the winding roads leading to Glanmore Lake. The focal length of my vision, synchronised so inextricably with my balance, created such feelings of nausea that I had to quit the woods after one or two attempts. I only had very rudimentary spectacles for seeing things and I clearly wasn't ready.

I tried the indoor swimming pool at the Great Southern, but my specs kept fogging up. Often I couldn't see a blessed thing, delighted nevertheless that I could swim. I had a couple of whole-body massages from the masseuse and felt my aching muscles respond like dried-up sponges, soaking up the massage-oil and stuff. My muscles ached for the welcome rejuvenation that only massage gave me.

Sometimes, after a light lunch in the hotel lounge, I sat back and dozed off, like an octogenarian. The incredible tiredness, which is part and parcel of stroke, had turned me into a snoring geriatric.

Winter was fast approaching; the sun had gone off for a cold shower and nature had pulled up its duvet for the Long Sleep. All the moist, earthy smells and sounds of birds were typical of Kerry and very consoling to the weary walker. I was becoming accustomed to the inclines and the terrain on my daily walking excursions.

It felt marvellous even to be able to stumble along the

equidistant four-mile Rosdohan and Oysterbed journeys. Although I was using my walking-stick almost like a crutch, to keep myself upright and steady, I felt very nervous every time a truck or car passed by, in case I ambled out into its path. However, I persevered; thankfully, the inbuilt determination to make it back towards normality knew no limitations.

ZERO POINT ONE SIX

TEN

Pain and Gain

'Picture the scene – you've just survived a combination of spectacular pain, unbelievable stress, gargantuan effort, tremendous joy and stunning relief. Way, way beyond anything you've experienced in your life before . . . .'

(Quote from a women's magazine, 1999)

In return, you might expect a standing ovation and genuine approval for such an incredible achievement. I am referring, of course, to that wondrous performance of women every time they give birth. Instead of being pampered and fussed over, as they should be (soccer players regularly are), they are generally dispatched as rapidly as possible from maternity hospitals, to ensure that the assembly line of newborn life doesn't suffer any hiccoughs.

I had never been involved in anything as earth-shattering as childbirth and wasn't prematurely turfed out of anywhere; nevertheless, I did feel fairly pleased with myself for having conquered my own mountain, and was content to share the event with even a few people.

After an eventful break in Kerry, we came home secure in the

knowledge that I could at least walk on my own, after a fashion, and could be expected back after each excursion without a distraught Mandy having to check with the local hospitals or the police! Now, though, I began to walk almost daily, determined to continue my rehabilitation, just as Professor O'Brien had advised me. I was relying then unbelievably heavily on his professional help.

I looked forward to all the walking, if not quite with alacrity, then with the ready acceptance of its absolute necessity, even to braving both the elements and the dim light on lousy mornings.

Simply wearing a ski-cap and gloves, a warm tracksuit and sporting the aluminium walking-stick, I struck out with hope on a three-mile walk. I welcomed that quietness of the first pre-Christmas period. Rainwater swelled the rivers, turning streams into torrents, waterfalls into roaring volcano-like eruptions, and left pools and lakes all over the place.

I was delighted to meet many old (and new) faces on these jaunts, greeting each other like long-lost friends. Their interest in my well-being helped a lot, making me realise what a lucky camper I was. It was always a tonic for me to stop and shoot the breeze with neighbours for a while; it made me feel even more in the land of the living.

It nevertheless felt incongruous, and rather sad, to be trundling along familiar routes that I had cycled before and jogged around with my friend Rambeau, now dead and buried in our front garden. Just in case you're wondering, Rambeau *was* our dog. He was having breakfast with me one morning when a sudden 'attack' aged him dramatically, transforming him almost instantaneously from a superb animal into a pitiful specimen. He died a half-hour later at the vet's. They diagnosed a ruptured spleen; he bled to death rapidly and painlessly. That was a year before my stroke.

I brought him home, travelling along all the familiar roads we had jogged along together, for one last time. I then buried him on our front lawn, in Liverpool Football Club hat, with my boots beside his head. Even though friends later replaced him with Rommel, another magnificent German Shepherd, who has also become a family member, I still miss Rambeau a lot, like a child, and regularly look at his portrait on the wall which we had commissioned a few years earlier.

Back in those carefree times, cycling and jogging weren't actually conducive to leisurely chats with the locals, and I did miss out hugely; but walking at a respectable pace was correcting all that. Take your time but hurry up! It normally took me just under an hour to walk the three-mile route and I felt good about that; but now with meeting people regularly it often took an extra five or ten minutes.

I began to take Buffy, our sole road-friendly Jack Russell, with me on an extension lead. She had often gone on runs with me before. She was great company, loving the freedom; but whenever she walked on my inside on the lead as cars approached it was all I could do to stop myself from falling on top of her. It certainly made me more careful about my balance; she looked up at me constantly, her eyes puzzled and worried, probably saying to herself, 'What in the name of all that's holy is wrong with yer man?'

I alternated this walk with another of four miles, just for a change of scenery; this latter route meandered quietly between a golf club and a stud farm. I had begun to visit a physiotherapist, who gave me a series of exercises to do when I was out walking. Since they all involved my legs only, and didn't make me look stupid, I felt relaxed about doing them in the open, holding on to a gate for balance even if someone happened to come upon me. These exercises greatly helped my balance, but my eyesight was again playing tricks with me and my specs urgently needed major adjustment.

The conifers were now the only green trees on my walks; all the other trees were bare, apart from the odd Douglas Fir. They looked like rows of waving hands, the tallest of which seemed to be shaking their fists in anger at the sky. I was reminded of the

life-size sculpture I had seen in Rotterdam years earlier, of a man with no heart, yelling out at the sky in a primordial scream. It signified for me that the heart of Rotterdam had been bombed by the Nazis during the Second World War, and that *that* particular sculpture served as a constant reminder. It was more dramatic even than that incredibly expressive painting *The Scream* by Edvard Munch and conveyed the same meaning. In a similar way the accusatory trees now reminded nature, even though it had closed up shop for the winter's sleep, not to forget them when the reawakening in the spring started the whole cycle of life all over again.

In a peculiar way, I felt that my walking, though flawed at that time, was crucial, as if reminding life itself that I used to be an athlete once, and wished dearly to get much better again as I ploughed the weary journey back towards normality. First, I had to get my defective eyes looked at straightaway. I visited my old friend, Dr Michael Browne, ophthalmic surgeon extraordinaire in his Tallaght Eyecentre, for a 60,000-mile check-up on the old eyes; he confirmed that I was ready for the next improvement to help me see things more clearly.

When I got the new eyepieces, I could virtually feel my eye muscles being strained back into their correct alignment; I could discern objects with far greater clarity and even the corner-of-my-eye vision presented none of the previous difficulties. My confidence grew as I began to see life more clearly. I was feeling less and less of an invalid.

However, while I was making great headway on my own personal level, I knew that something was compelling me towards upsetting both Mandy and Emma – holding back the development of our ongoing relationship. We wanted to get things right, desperately, and I was working like hell at that.

My developing independence was obviously suiting us all though, after all the customer is nearly always right and I was the seller. I just *had* to get it right; I'd no other choice.

ELEVEN

Front-seat Driver

I am normally a very voluble passenger in my own car; I find fault with nearly everything. Is that a natural phenomenon? The odd time, though, whenever I've been driven in someone else's, I've always enjoyed it. I am definitely not a back-seat driver.

But when Mandy was driving me, up until about April 1997, hardly anything she did was right! 'Stop there; pass here; go now; watch out; brake hard; for God's sake speed up – are you on a tour or something?' and a litany of other unnecessary hints punctuated every drive. How I ever thought that she needed my constant advice to 'help' her baffles me now.

I could sense that she and Emma winced whenever I began to get into full stride and gradually withdrew into themselves, assuming a feigned nonchalance as they tried to ignore my ridiculous prattle. It must have been mental torture for them to take me for drives, knowing what to expect. However, try as I might, I couldn't help myself – and I did try. I hated being an insufferable know-all.

Do husbands normally behave like that when their beloveds are driving them? I doubt it. I'm sure the odd row is a fairly normal occurrence, but *every* time? I would have hated to be married to *me* during that crazy period. At any rate, I was getting

on Mandy and Emma's nerves, so before murder became a necessary solution, I decided that the situation could be retrieved if I began to drive by myself – and the sooner the better.

I had passed the mandatory written/oral driving examination during my recovery at the Rehab Hospital and Michael Browne assured me that I was fine – and for driving too. In fact there are people probably driving around, unconcerned and free of guilt, nearly deaf, dumb and blind. A body that had been stuffed and mounted could perhaps wangle a driving licence somehow.

Conor Devine, our GP, filled in the required questionnaire on my health status for insurance purposes, and I was ready to roll. Balance was not a problem for me while sitting down, or driving; I experienced unsteadiness only when I was standing or walking.

Beginning to drive all over again was like the very first time, except that now I could handle the car and its controls much better than during my earliest attempts as a callow teenager. I had to relearn many things: like an appreciation of speed, how quickly other cars were going, the capacities of my own steed, distances, when to pull back in and stay put or when to pass. It felt strange for quite a while, not actually worrying, but 'different', as the old familiar touches and feelings gradually returned and I became a better judge – and a surer driver. I loved the feeling of freedom that it gave me, and the breaks it gave my family *from me* were worth all the effort; Mandy and Emma gradually slipped back to driving about in their own red Jeep again.

I drove around for miles as if some force was compelling me to wallow in the new-found freedom. The views along the country lanes and byroads of Kildare, Wicklow and Dublin were the tonic that would help propel my recovery even further, as I travelled in open-eyed wonderment, like a dog suddenly confronted by two telegraph poles!

I had to exercise extreme care, coming on to main roads particularly, to avoid a blind spot whenever I looked out of the corner of either eye. Whereas before a quick glance was enough to take in anything approaching from either side, I now had to pause and make sure that the road was clear both ways. The eye-correlation between the rearview mirror and those at the sides caused me considerable frustration; it took almost two years of post-haemorrhage driving before I felt confident enough to take in all three at a glance, like before.

Those early problems of co-ordination with the three mirrors often caused severe consternation, especially at night on the three-lane carriageway leading south from Dublin. Passing a slowcoach hogging the middle lane, on his inside, may be illegal, but it was fine by me; however, finding *myself* driving at a reasonable pace in the middle lane was disconcerting whenever I was passed simultaneously by two madmen on either side.

So I was delighted to be able to drive around on my own; pretty soon the competitive edge emerged and I felt compelled to take on younger blokes, showing them that Mick and his coupé could still match the best, or so I believed. I felt like the husband given a book for Christmas on *How to be boss in your own home*, only to find that his wife wouldn't let him read it. Fortunately for us all, Mandy put a break on my competitive tendencies.

I find that driving under the influence of water nowadays feels peculiar, but is a real boon at police checkpoints – I almost feel cheeky; but I remember what an old police mate of mine in Bristol, the wily John Broadbelt, always said, in his West Country accent, 'Remember, Moike, don't bloody draw attention to y'reself.' It was good advice, especially coming from a copper; he should know, he drank enough with me whenever we met up. He's still going strong, too.

With the novelty of driving I felt a more complete person again and didn't have to depend on anyone else. It was as if my life had begun falling back gradually into its former cycle and all the 'new', exciting vistas and experiences soon became normal.

But I feel now that I *have* experienced a renewed, even an exalted appreciation of nature from my car window. Whether it was a function of driving once more or the confidence born of freedom from booze, I don't altogether know, but I couldn't care less. I adore driving now, the further the better, and we three have found our peaceful lifestyles restored.

All in all, I have gained a lot since my days at Beaumont, and so I should! It feels funny now to be driving back there to see friends, and also to the Rehab Hospital, and meeting the staff members. I can't help thinking that only a few short years ago I was awkwardly learning how to drive a wheelchair.

TWELVE

Getting the Brain in Gear

Once I could, but I wouldn't,
Now I would, but I can't.

The late Rev. David Walsh, a kindly man, whom I've known since childhood in Currow village, where I was born, inveigled me, successfully, with these fairly stark words out of the hazards of lethargy and the clutches of early excesses – especially of food and of drink. It was 1973.

He shocked me into understanding that if I let life pass me by, when I could do something to change its inexorable course, the time would eventually come when I wouldn't physically be able to do what I really wanted – I would become like a couch potato in front of a TV screen. Perhaps wearing a trendy tracksuit and a pair of top-of-the-range runners to make me feel athletic! Anyway, his timely intervention propelled me back into rugby football again and a new prospectus of playing, influencing, selecting and coaching – right up to the top of the international mound – opened up.

In 1968 I had retired, aged twenty-eight, from rugby, 'learned' to drink and allowed inactivity and the good life to seduce me. While my sports life flourished, the other side, the darker,

camouflaged, social side of me, continued on its slow, invisible, downward spiral, completely contrary to what I actually believed was happening to me. The brain haemorrhage finally halted the wild downhill *slalom*, making me realise that 'Now that I would, I can't.'

Currow village is a remarkable place; I won't bore you, except to tell you that four Irish Rugby internationals went to school there, including three British Lions: Moss Keane, Michael Galwey and myself. My brother Tom was the fourth.

What is equally extraordinary is that rugby was *never* played in Currow, it being a Gaelic football village, the game which we all grew up playing. Being a native, I'm always proud to be from there; naturally I'll never forget it. Moss gave Galwey very pertinent advice before his first game against France: 'Forget about the ball for the first half-hour,' advised Moss, 'and concentrate instead on yer man; that's how to make your mark on the French!'

The poor old French must have reckoned that yet another madman had been selected by the Irish; a bit like Wales's 'outhalf factories' we must have had a quarry-full of maniacs. Paddies with attitude.

One day, in the spring of 1999, as I was having a light breakfast before my usual walk, I looked out of the patio door and could clearly see Miss Muffet, our roan Shetland, standing almost at the crest of the hill field that intercepted our view of the picturesque Wicklow mountains. Dwarfing Lucy Locket, a six-month Shetland foal, by a full two inches, Miss Muffet gazed around her at the heavily pregnant sheep who were munching nonchalantly away.

Muffet, to my imagination, looked like a pontiff, pointing out to them where they should stand and arrange themselves, uncannily reminiscent of a wise cricket captain rearranging his forces, particularly his outfielders, with every new change of batsman. After a while the docile sheep seemed to adjust themselves, though their indifference conveyed that they couldn't really be bothered. They presented a quiet picture of passive acquiescence.

It was rather hard to believe, as I drank in this natural order of life everywhere around me, that it was only a short three or so years earlier when the strings attaching my tenuous hold on life almost snapped forever. It has forced me into becoming a much more organised person, not unlike Miss Muffet's woolly friends. It certainly helped me in my struggles along the oft-weary journey back towards being well, and, like Miss Muffet, I had to become a resourceful organiser. Self-help and all that.

Pondering on the unpredictable future that stretched ahead for us brain-haemorrhage victims, I wholeheartedly agreed first of all with the Beatles when they sang, 'Love is all you need', back in 1967. We could do the rest ourselves; for so long as we were loved and wanted and encouraged to help ourselves, anything was possible!

I have often been asked a lot of very pertinent questions by many people who have experienced, like me, the varying effects of stroke, of car accidents, head injuries, heart by-pass surgery and indeed of anything that could alter their lives. In addition their close family members continually seek help and advice, all trying to adjust to their relatives' recovery and rehabilitation into society, as they come to grips with the much-changed circumstances.

I suppose, because I was able to motivate international rugby players, that people felt that I may have ready-made words of advice for them. I would love to oblige and I hope the following makes some sense.

At the outset, I can honestly say that I had to poke around for answers myself; I had no one who could fully explain to me what to expect in the aftermath of stroke. I had been unlucky in a lifestyle that encouraged my appetites, and extremely fortunate to have been a motivated person in the first place – an 'achiever' in popular parlance. Of course I had been heavily involved for much of my life with equally motivated people and was well used to

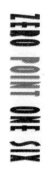

setting goals for myself and others. The various prompts of my sports days stood by me now when I was in most need of help, acting as my guidedog during the early dark days of recovery, when I felt that almost everything was stacked against me.

The psychology inherent in coaching serious international players is really demanding, and it had required a high level of commitment from me. I was only too delighted to become involved with the players anyway as they were such a superb group; still, the route to the pursuit of excellence was strewn with many disappointments, interspersed with times of incredible satisfaction and enjoyment.

The fact that it was a true labour of love back then before rugby became professional, and that I had a busy consultancy veterinary practice and a developing business, added extra focus and real fun to the whole exercise. I needed to be very organised to fit coaching into a crowded schedule, and I compart-mentalised my working life to accommodate everything. The physical commitments of training schedules and actual playing were relatively easy to orchestrate into an agenda; it was the *mental* part of the whole equation that occupied so many waking hours. I regularly dreamed rugby, too.

Planning was essential. The whole exercise was real fun though, and my commitment to the players was absolute. I loved, admired and trusted them. The fact that it was unpaid, fitting into my professional and business life as it did, created such an exciting 'buzz'. At the end of five glorious years with Leinster and three with Irish rugby I was sad to be leaving such incredible blokes, but financially I could not afford to be involved in coaching for any longer. Anyway, I would never have done it for money – to be anyone's paid hand.

That statement might seem somewhat arrogant, but, viewed from my position, I then had an all-embracing veterinary practice and a business to run, and since my involvement with rugby was personal, private and strictly in accordance with the amateur ethos of the time, it just didn't arise that I would ever need to make a career of coaching. Anyway, I was too steeped in this ethos to become anything else – I just switched off.

Different strokes for different folks obviously. However, spare time very nearly became full time. That was the past; now, at home, with the support system of the Rehab Hospital eliminated, I was left to flounder, motivating nobody but myself. This time around, everything was totally different; I now had to motivate myself alone. Nothing was easy. I had to convince myself that I would get better, and I wouldn't have bet the family heirlooms on that particular outcome.

I had to try to ignore most of my afflictions, something like the rains of summer weather in Ireland – treating all my current imperfections as merely temporary; I was driven instead to concentrate on the positive things to which I could look forward, while keeping negatives in abeyance. But where should I start?

Well, I had to accept that I was utterly changed, a different person. The person that was had gone forever, and the present shapeless form of what I could become filled me with a formidable trepidation and a deep suspicion of what lay ahead. Funnily enough though, it also fired me with an insatiable curiosity and a steely determination to make it, whatever 'it' was. It was like playing rugby for Ireland or the British Lions all over again, but the challenge this time was far more serious – and deep down it frightened me.

I blindly lived in hope in those early days of my escape to the outside world, even though I was confined to a wheelchair. I had certainly been dealt a poor hand, but I had to play it as best I could. I reckon now, despite the futile hope my dismal situation suggested, that I was never more determined in my life; but even then it was a serious struggle.

The conscious will to get better battled constantly with the powerful negative promptings of my subconscious, to settle somewhere in peace and quiet, and to avoid all the difficult regimes threatening to stretch out in front of me; the comfort zone tempted me.

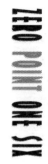

However, mercifully, the overpowering desire to make it back kept bringing me back to the scene of the 'accident', whispering words of encouragement to me. The future was of far more relevance now than the past; former memories had to be consigned to left-luggage lockers for the time being. Subconsciously I was still a reluctant traveller, trying to bask in the memories of former glory.

Surely if we knew for certain what lay in store for us, we would either be bored silly, or else become too lazy to try hard enough. However, I decided to go for it, to put aside the interruptions of the past for later enjoyment. I had to ignore the major roads at first, travelling instead on the less predictable byways.

Like giving up smoking years before, I had to prepare myself mentally; I needed to be brutally honest with myself to be aware of what I was and what I could become, I needed to analyse my current abilities – which wasn't too difficult to do (I could just about go to the toilet by myself, and shave) – and those that I desperately craved to recapture.

To achieve anything of worth, I felt that my mind and body needed to work in harmony; the mental and physical commitment had to be absolute. I knew from my former life that if my commitment became diluted in any way, I would achieve only partial success. This was focusing with a capital 'F'. It became my eight-letter word!

I began to like my new self; I realised that I had been a competitor in most things I did, and that I liked winning, hated losing. I felt *comfortable* about being blindly ambitious for myself. The newness of everything, the changed reality, suggested that I had to reassess my capacity to be objective about the altered facets of life, forcing myself to understand exactly what was driving me. In short, I had to go out on a limb for myself; first I needed to venture on to the greasy pole of uncertainty with my mind, and then follow it with all the physical abilities I could muster. That's how way out I had to become – me against the world!

Like most sports' coaches, I was scared that I wouldn't do enough to surmount my own deficiencies, that I might settle for a cosy existence. After all, I was stuck in a wheelchair; all progress had to be carefully charted and well directed.

I decided early on to move straight from the wheelchair to the aluminium walking-stick, short-circuiting the journey by avoiding the Zimmer frame as much as possible. I hardly ever had to use it. Cutting out that step did wonders for my self-confidence.

The cult of self-preservation, that inbuilt drive to succeed that all humans possess, becomes merged with the absolute determination to proceed regardless, becoming like a long-playing video of your life, wherein most of the major happenings suddenly become important milestones, in your time of most need.

Something else also happens – all those other not-so-readily-recalled experiences, which you felt had been deeply buried, happening such a long time ago, suddenly become important and assume a central role in your new life. It is as if all those little incidentals coalesced until they formed one giant snowball of positiveness: a prop to the main drive to improve.

I was aware that I was lucky in many ways – just to be alive for one; to have given up tobacco and been forced to quit the booze were big pluses for me, but also being able to reflect on a period of extreme motivation in my former life helped enormously.

My younger brother Tom often remarked to me that all the daft things I did as a kid, like picking wild blackberries, stealing apples from orchards, fishing in the rivers, chasing rabbits around the bogs of Kerry, playing football and the wild pursuits of the young who are lucky to be brought up in the countryside, now became welded into a powerful driving force. They helped along my physical side by providing the latent stamina that I urgently needed, proving that former habits do not die that easily. I am sure that many people have similar experiences, and can draw on them in times of real need, to synchronise with the

bigger positives that will jointly help them towards becoming well again.

I felt quite certain, once I had pointed myself in the right general direction, that I had to have the goals I craved irrevocably set in stone; I just couldn't allow myself to settle for anything less. I couldn't let *me* down. I was unable to blame anybody else anyhow.

In order to reach my goal, I had to strive continually to ensure that all thoughts about recovery were realistic, yet positive (or vice versa), that I would need to summon all my abilities and energy to complete even the simplest of tasks, like walking every single day, and, amid all this seriousness, I had to preserve both a sense of balance and of humour to see the funny side of life – to laugh at myself, even though there wasn't much to laugh about; certainly not early on!

It is most probable that a sense of humour preserves your sanity when you have given up the booze, and try to improve, ensuring that you do not develop into a morose shadow of what you were before. The challenge is quietly and persistently waiting to be taken up, to demonstrate to everyone around you that abstinence will not alter your appreciation of fun and that you do not need to become immersed in drink to be as good a companion as you formerly were. I was lucky there too; it worked for me and I had genuinely been afraid of becoming a bore.

When I consider it all now, I know that I had to perpetually envisage myself as I wanted to be, the new me, and to aim, to the exclusion of all else, at that specific state. In short, I had to rebuild myself. My wife and family could help me with the capsule of their love and support but I had to slog it out all by myself – to give them (and me) something to cling on to.

Of course all this placed a fair old burden on self-belief, but that never let me down, thank the Lord, even when I felt like quitting. I kept telling myself that I had the commitment and the sense of pride to write my own script, to set out my own personal goals. I had to think for myself. Something intrinsic drove me on compulsively, like a guardian angel might, to think outside myself, to keep my ambition threshold raised towards a very high objective. I was extremely lucky that I had been accustomed to dream regularly about favourable outcomes during my rugby-coaching days; it helped me enormously now to contemplate the future me, to realise what I would become, and to articulate it to my wife, my family and my friends. Self-talk equated to self-help.

It is ridiculously ironical, when you can hardly stand up straight without the support of a wheelchair or a Zimmer frame, to be dreaming about walking around normally and mingling with your friends. Although negative thoughts never occurred in any serious way with me, other than the normal doubts that we all get waylaid by sometimes, I did not let self-pity enter my mind, not even once.

It may even sound incongruous, but life became one big dream machine, like horse-racing or sport. I constantly imagined myself in various situations, each one better than the other. Everything seemed larger than normal, much more relevant, and the previous adversities that used to niggle me I regarded now as somebody else's problem – mere peripherals. A new perspective on life took over, and the central driving force was to get back to normal.

I had the freedom to follow a charted course, like a railway line, but nevertheless the challenge was huge. Self-help, self-propulsion, both helped me to maintain and even increase the pace, withstand more pain and imaginary indignities, and pursue more and more intensity in the daily struggles. I had to attack all the negatives that kept trying to interfere, to consign question marks, anxieties and any smidgen of self-doubt to the waste heap. I had to remain entirely positive and concentrated, and it certainly worked for me.

Of course, like everybody else, I came across many different problems en route, and I had to learn to adapt, just like I had to

ZERO POINT ONE SIX

do as a coach. For example, I felt the pounds piling on again about October 1997, sixteen months after the stroke, affecting my walking and my balance. I followed the Nutron Diet and shed about fourteen kilos. This method of weight-reduction involves submitting a blood sample to the Nutron Clinic so that you can be advised what foods to avoid and which to indulge your cravings. Clients are provided with a simple, personalised pocket chart which they try to adhere to; they are weighed weekly by the clinic's personnel and given lymphatic electro-massage and the like to help shake off the pounds. It was a success, too.

My feet and calf muscles ached from all the walking. I decided to keep on plodding along, but began a course of reflexology, with Sarah, who massaged my feet, thoroughly, once a week for a few months. Resting actually does nothing for most complaints; all the massage and the walking helped to sort out the discomfort.

Gradually I developed a new identity as I shed the old one and life became consumed with a renewed self-belief, a confident sense of purpose. The invalid was being transformed into the new me and in the process I learned to redefine where I was going and how I might get there; of course, it is often more important to realise how you actually won than why you did not achieve what you set out to do.

The old SAS motto 'who dares wins' was very appropriate in my circumstances, even though I was afraid to dare too much. Every now and again I received a sharp reminder that I was flawed, and that no matter how well I became, I would never be the same again. No England on wet afternoons.

While in previous times, for all of us in Irish rugby in the 1980s, it was the performance itself, the manner of winning, the attendant hype, the support of the public, the approval of the commentators, and the roar of the crowd that lived on in our memory, things were much more private and personal now. No crowds; no standing ovations. Just me and the elements.

So, as I strove towards becoming better, using all my will-power and talents, I realised what a small cog in a giant wheel I actually was; but I know now that self-belief and self-help are twin travelling companions, always. And they both helped me enormously.

If success seems to be slow in coming, almost evading you, and you're becoming frustrated, all I can say is that this happened to me, too, and I often had to wait a while longer than I had anticipated. So don't worry; don't despair; getting better will always take its own good time. Everything has a sort of inevitability about it, a predictability, hasn't it?

I know now that I have made a highly satisfactory recovery, but I wished that I hadn't experienced that particular career move in the first place. However, John Murphy and Ann Keane had taught me well, preparing me for the struggle and a new beginning.

In the final analysis, we were all lucky as a family that I made it back to something like I used to be. As the famous American football coach Vince Lombardi once remarked: 'The difference between a successful person and others is not a lack of strength, not a lack of knowledge, but rather a lack of will.' That is so, so apt.

Since you only get one chance to make a good *first* impression, it is absolutely vital not to leave any pool unfished, nothing to chance, as you begin the strange, lonely journey back to wholeness. Nothing comes easy, and all the lone efforts during our struggles must become fused with our mental yearnings until they become as one.

I have always reckoned that the human spirit often defies the odds, displaying incredible resilience. The famous American sports commentator was right when he observed, 'The man who wins may have been counted out several times, but he didn't hear the referee.' Amen, Olé and whatever you're havin' to drink yourself. Winning was, and is, the only worthwhile thing. Bill Shankley was dead right. I was fortunate to coach a superb group

ZERO POINT ONE SIX

of Irish players from 1984 to 1987. That was a magic time. As I was pushing a very late Trevor Ringland and Keith Crossan on to the bus for Murrayfield, just before the first championship game with Scotland in 1985, Gerald Davies, a mate from the 1968 Lions Rugby Tour in South Africa and one of the world's all-time great wing threequarters, now corresponding for *The Times*, said, 'Mick, a quick word.'

'Sure, Gerald.'

'What did your boys learn from watching the [Cliff Morgan] video of the Welsh crowning years?'

(We were literally amazed by the incredible play of the Welsh, but I wouldn't admit it to Gerald.) 'Gerald, old son, we learnt that if fifteen thick Welsh miners could play football like that, then so could fifteen super intelligent Paddies!'

I believe he printed this joke. However, though I didn't mean anything like that, we did have a belief in that particular Irish squad that anything was possible and that performance was king. It certainly was critical for a rather compromised me from now on.

Closer to home, I was lying in bed in hospital, having just awoken from my month's sleep, when I noticed Willie Anderson sitting quietly beside my bed. Willie captained Ireland in the late 1980s and was always a superb athlete. I loved coaching him.

Willie doesn't normally talk much, so we both exchanged short sentences of question and answer.

'What's the word among the lads about me?' I asked.

'Oh, you're finished,' he said laconically.

That was the motivation I needed. No wonder Willie is such a good coach nowadays: his team, Dungannon, won the A.I.B., All Ireland League, this season; in brilliant fashion I must add.

THIRTEEN

Chastity Belts for Head Cases

I had always believed that vertigo had been invented by Alfred Hitchcock and had only ever appeared in his own movies. Obviously I was way off the mark.

I had first attended a particular physiotherapist on the advice of the neurologist, whom Dr Eóin O'Brien had arranged for me to see in Beaumont Hospital, sometime around March 1997. I had a peculiar complaint then: I was physically able to walk, albeit unsteadily, but not only was my head buzzing chronically, it also felt wooden-like, and vertigo was playing havoc with my balance.

I felt that I could beat the whole world when I was lying down, as in bed; but getting up triggered the whole unwelcome process, and I began to feel that I could fall over at any time, even on the short trip to the armchair. Merely sitting up in the armchair produced its own discomfort and confusion; and whenever I stood up I felt that I would be better off back in Beaumont again. It was horrible, and worrying.

It is difficult to describe, but it was as if my whole head was encased in a giant plastic bubble, confined and constrained, like the man in the iron mask; it was constricting me, like chastity belts must have done in the days of the Crusaders. Whoever had the infernal key had chucked it away.

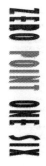

ZERO POINT ONE SIX

145

It was reckoned that my disorientation could be caused by any number of things, like getting up too fast, or perhaps by hydrocephalus (water on the brain). The neurologist eliminated all the usual suspects, to my relief but still obvious bafflement, and recommended that I undertake a course of physiotherapy, to help my balance.

Vertigo had suddenly broken into my life, shattering my carefully crafted script for getting better, ensnaring any attempts at normality and almost swamping my will-power. Any determination that I had painstakingly built up to escape from the shackles of serfdom experienced by the invalid, which subarachnoid haemorrhage regularly imposes, and to embrace the free pursuits of life on the outside, took a fair old battering. It struggled along with a decided limp until about June 1997, when happily I was able to force myself to begin walking again in fresh surroundings, on holiday in Kerry. The medics, the physiotherapy, the resting, the walking and the eye fine-tuning all helped me in the end.

Whenever I think of walking in Kerry, I envisage a profusion of fuchsias in every hedge and roadside, forming great swathes of growth along the hills and valleys. Their little red bells, with their purple lining and green strikers, as in a church, hang like pendulous earrings, dancing in the breeze – a sea of nodding heads.

It was very different from the last time I went; I could cycle then. I could just about walk now, and I had barely started on the Nutron Diet. It felt like going off on holiday to one of those weight-control health farms, but at our holiday home on the Connor Pass there was no one watching, no one counting the calories except ourselves – and we weren't to be conned.

I lost seven or eight pounds during the holidays – a wholly unusual occurrence for me. Apart from being off the booze, I didn't feel in any way deprived, or on rations. But I had to work at it.

I drank the four regulation pints of water a day, and if they had been dishing out sporrans with Irish crests on them, I could have piddled for Ireland. Alongside all this, the onerous walking improved considerably. Up Kerry.

Conor Devine, our GP, called often, establishing that my blood pressure was a bit high, but not seriously, and that I was suffering from *nystagmus*; in other words, my eyes did not follow an object across their line of vision smoothly, to each corner, as they should; instead, they moved in a series of jerks. Time would cure that, Conor said. I felt fortunate, perversely enough, that one eye wasn't so good-looking that the other one couldn't stop looking at it!

I rested at home for a couple of weeks and after a few trips to the physiotherapist the leg exercises not only helped my walking but also my balance. When I was shaving I could at least stand up, even though I couldn't see my beard growth clearly without squinting through one eye. I wasn't up to using the shower though; I couldn't step over the side of the bath or stand up unaided under the water jets. However, I became an expert on baths, keeping the hot water topped up, adjusting the taps with my toes.

––––––––––––––

Backing up a bit on the whole time-scale, from about November 1996 right through to the following March, I had luckily been making great gains at walking, talking and sleeping. A positive mental attitude generally kept most shadows at bay, and it seemed that recovery would be progressive, steady and relatively smooth. Unfortunately, as usual, fate took an armful, instead of the more customary hand, and things ceased to sail along on their anticipated course. Simplicity was for someone else, obviously.

Vertigo had struck with almost a fury, suggesting that Alfred Hitchcock was still weaving his magic from beyond the crematorium. Any intentions I had entertained of improving my balance evaporated rapidly, changing abruptly into a struggle to pick up the piecemeal threads again.

Thankfully, the plastic bubble gradually and finally faded away, leaving in its wake vivid reminders of its effects on me, and the ghosts of its presence – and just vertigo.

When I couldn't bear the idea of walking, in April/May 1997, I had begun driving as a compensatory mechanism: 'If I can't walk, then I'll drive,' I reasoned.

Mercifully, I had started getting on a lot better with Mandy and Emma, far more normal now that I had stopped getting on their nerves, which must have been hypersensitively strung out by this stage. I was still dominated by the cantankerousness associated with brain haemorrhage (why had nobody ever warned me?) and found myself behaving in ways that were decidedly alien to my normal pattern: hypercritical and self-centred were two 'attributes' not normally identified with me previously, but had now become hallmarks.

I knew exactly what was going on. I tried in vain to revert back to how I was before, but I couldn't help myself from saying and doing stupid things: Mandy and Emma continually seemed to *need* my advice and help! The water was always too hot, or the TV too loud, or the dogs too frisky. Nothing was in its right place; I found fault with everything.

Of course, knowing how my family and all my friends must have felt probably put an extra burden on me, too. I almost but didn't say, 'What's the point of going on?' But it really did bother me, intensely, that I seemed compelled to annoy everyone so much. It must have been testing *their* patience too and I *was* desperately trying to handle what I hoped was a temporary aberration. 'I won't stay like this, stuck in a deep rut of a time warp, from now on, will I?' I asked myself. I hoped that it wouldn't be so, and took all the precautions I could to make sure.

Looking back on it all now, I suppose that a great many people were hurting to realise that I was so utterly changed, reduced to this awkward state of thorny human. And so, while any resolutions to get walking again had to be sidelined for a while, I changed mental direction at roughly the same time, channelling all my energies into driving. 'Any port in a storm', as the sailor was reputed to have said. It really was a huge psychological boost and one we all needed, desperately, and in the nick of time, too. Before I changed for the better, Mandy and Emma must have wondered if I would remain a grumpy, irrational irritant forever.

Some driving experiences did linger in my memory though; they still accompany me everywhere I travel: after mastering the intricacies of the car, I was always extremely grateful and happy to see so many beautiful places on revisits, knowing that, had I died, I wouldn't have seen them again. It must be something like being given one year of life, with the threat of an incurable disease hanging over everything and everyone, trying to pack as much activity as possible into those twelve precious months.

I constantly feel like that now; I love stopping for even a while at some breathtaking landscapes and seaviews, mountains, valleys. I'm very glad that I'm still around to appreciate it all.

However, pretty soon the urge to walk again, the challenge to master all my imperfections became so great, that not even driving could substitute for it. *Not* walking had become quite an issue; walking looked like the answer. Fortunately, the bubble had faded and I was just left with vertigo to handle as best I could. Inactivity, funnily enough, had helped to relieve and finally overcome the chastity-belt phenomenon, but only the physical activity of walking and the balancing exercises helped me to make the necessary progress with imbalance and vertigo.

Soon, other niggling deficiencies manifested themselves as I gradually returned to something like normality. Not only was I a bit wobbly for example around the house or at the office, or in the shops, but I also found to my dismay that looking upwards, with my face receiving the full force of the bathroom shower, caused severe problems: a feeling of blackout, where the back of my head went numb, occurred regularly. Eventually I was even

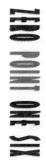

ZERO POINT ONE SIX

waiting for it to happen. It was like the feeling I got when my head fell too quickly on to the pillow; or when I banged my skull off the hard concrete as a child. A ringing numbness made me stop, as if frozen in situ, but quite quickly the disorientation and discomfort would pass. It must have been my injured brain telling me to take it easy; that it was too soon for me to expect miracles. The *only* miracles would be the habitual things we do in our daily lives, but I had to be much more careful now, and do even simple things more gradually.

I found it impossible, without toppling over, to stand with one foot roughly in front of the other, as in measuring off the dimensions of a room; and I still do, over five years later, even though it has dramatically improved. It seems as if the brain cells controlling that particular function have been damaged irreparably and can no longer operate successfully. Perhaps time will heal that deficiency too.

An interesting feature (I'm a mine of useless information) was that I found I could not balance on one leg to step into my trousers, unless I had a support. I often thought of Ronald Reagan, who, as the seventy-odd-year-old US president, boasted that he could get into his socks while balancing on one foot. It has taken me three years to master that magnificent achievement and I can't help wondering, what earthly difference does it make anyway?

Another zone of discomfort was digging in the garden, or bending down repeatedly to clean up after the dogs on the lawn – this always caused me severe headaches and nausea. Similarly, washing the car, a simple task normally, but the continued, rapid movement up and down, cleaning the sides or the wheels, caused me similar faintness. I often had to hold my head with the dizziness and pain. This has gradually disappeared now, yet again proving that, like watching a kettle boil, one can do very little to shorten the repair time. As with road rage, there is little to be gained by impatience. It is obviously far better to accept that some things are not under one's own control, and concentrate instead on those things on which one can improve.

Now over five years on, I still have slight problems whenever I try to turn around. I have also found it extremely difficult, even highly embarrassing, to negotiate steps: climbing on to a stage, or negotiating the stairs of a football stand. I am vastly improved now but back then I was always grateful for a helping hand or a handy railing.

I feel sure that rest would have done very little good in my case; I had to practise and practise to see any improvement. This worked for me, proving yet again that only perfect practice makes perfect, though in my case I always fell short of perfection.

Cycling in those early days of recovery was out of bounds. My balance was fine but the fear of having to find my footing at stops on major roads, or to halt suddenly, bothered me. I learned to cycle again around July 2000 and now adore the freedom and the feeling of being at peace with nature that it gives me.

In cycling, as with jogging, the sensation of 'running inside your head' always promoted progressive hormone-induced contentment, as the cares of the world faded away.

As I became used to the art of walking again, I drew inspiration from the tourists in passing cars and buses who seemed pleased to recognise a lone hiker. Normality forged an incredible impression on me. I was in heaven again; heaven on earth. I was at home on the Dingle Peninsula. It was good to be alive, back among the living. Mount Brandon stood guard over me.

It is often peculiar how the expected fails to occur according to plan, but, like the spider's web, it surreptitiously crops up out of the blue. A stroke often does that.

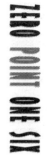

Depression was similar for me. However, during my time in Beaumont and the Rehabilitation Hospital I never received the slightest preview of this dreadful horror movie. Even for the first year or so of recovery at home I had been miraculously free of any major deviations of the mind; I was not impeded by any such obstacles to my plans for improvement.

I had received a surface level of counselling from a social worker in the Rehab Hospital about a week before I left. She was probably ideal for the many superficial problems, but any deeper analysis would naturally have required the services of a trained mind-doctor. But the shallows of the mind gradually yielded ground to the dark pools of depression; I soon felt as helpless as a cork bobbing around in a turbulent sea.

Mind you, despite being the subject of deep gloom and greyness, I never had any feelings of pessimism or suffered a lack of objectivity. I had honestly replied to the Social Welfare specialist in the Rehab around October 1996 that no, I didn't experience the customary depression associated with stroke; it was probably too soon anyway since July to have made itself manifest. Certainly it would have been a new experience for me – I had never felt depressed or inadequate at any time in my life, except perhaps momentarily following my 'coronary incident' in New Zealand in 1987.

I was extremely lucky once again not to have a wall of impossibility obstructing my recovery. Optimism was still the tune playing in my head, even if at times it was only a faint echo when circumstances conspired to thwart me: like, for example, the vertigo.

I knew where I wanted to go, but the getting there had suddenly lost its urgency. There seemed to be no great hurry. I felt useless and irrelevant, in a time warp where everybody seemed to move in slow motion. I felt that I'd get better eventually, and all the walking I'd done had worked wonders for my self-confidence and motivation, but even all that seemed irrelevant during the onslaught of depression.

A number of things had been gathering ominously, like storm clouds on the horizon. Jumbled up with them was a series of events that triggered off significant effects on me, making me hyperconscious of everything about mortality. Like, what the hell was the whole purpose?

Having returned home from Dingle, for example, we travelled down again almost immediately to the untimely burial of Davey Browne, the teenage son of our friends Hannah Mae and Ted. He had fallen a few hundred feet to his death from a cliff top as he was rescuing an injured seagull. It was devastating and has had an indelible effect on me since; as had the earlier death from cancer of the throat of my close friend and colleague Tony James.

Of far lesser import but still of significant impact were the deaths of hamster Lisa and our doggy pals Buffy and Mouse. Lisa and Buffy had reached the age where they would be taking their leave of this life anyway, but little Mouse was cruelly killed on the roadside near our home. I missed them all; Emma was devastated, and Mandy was intensely sad.

This relinquishing of the strands of life and the sad circumstances surrounding each event, seemed to play havoc with my will-power and perspective. Luckily I could read the signs and see things coming before I succumbed to the compulsion of depression.

The symptoms frightened me. Fortunately, I sought the timely advice of our GP. He saw all the signals as well, and prescribed a course of Cipramil tablets; a mild antidepressant. Basically they did the trick and I luckily got them before my resolve took a hammering. Acting in time helped me to refocus quickly, preventing pessimism from getting a toehold in my subconscious, but it was a narrow escape.

Then, in early 1999 my first father-in-law, farmer Vic Thompson, died of Alzheimer's in Penford, Somerset. I had always loved him; he and his wife Sybil had been such a positive influence on my growing up. His death forged its own impact on my depressive state of mind.

ZERO POINT ONE SIX

I have since learned that depression is actually part and parcel of the aftermath of brain haemorrhage. It is normally expected to occur sometime after the realisation of incapacity first hits one, and gradually begins to interfere with recuperation. However, in my case it was headed off at the pass.

It was still a frightening experience, possibly starting weeks or months before I saw the danger signs; then after the appropriate dosage rate became established the antidepressants began to work, making life look more enticing again.

It was surely an undeniable mistake that my family and I had received no forewarning that depression could happen and that it could be so devastating. Clearly, it was a glaring omission in the whole recuperation procedure, when a comprehensive package of discussion and written instructions should accompany every 'going home' patient.

Another psychological phenomenon to affect me, as with almost all stroke victims I believe, was extreme fatigue; sure, we all feel tired from time to time but this fatigue was like a debilitating illness. When one considers the bombardment that occurs to one's body during a stroke and the subsequent trauma, weight loss, deprivation and frustration, is it really any wonder that severe exhaustion sets in?

The exhaustion began noticeably when I finally came home from hospital and it seriously taxed my mental and physical resolve. I suppose it was nature's way of telling me to take things easier. Whatever the cause, the fatigue certainly made me feel unsteady now and again (even now) and I always know that tiredness is coming on if I begin to wobble a bit more when I walk.

I have accepted without frustration, or stroke rage, the twin-assaults to the system, realising full well that while depression and the feeling of less than usefulness are both natural phenomena, fatigue itself is that much easier to handle. It is important for victims to realise how inevitable both conditions are, but it is vital not to let depression gain any meaningful purchase on your fragile faculties.

As Mae West was reputed to have said, 'Whenever I'm faced with a choice of two evils, I always pick the one that I haven't tried before.' I've often felt like that; except that, for me, tiredness was normal, depression entirely new.

It was somewhat reminiscent of after the Lions v Rhodesia game in Salisbury in 1968: Willie John, Syd Millar and myself were chatting to the prime minister, Ian Smith, beside a barrel of Whitbread South Africa at a Salisbury party, when John (Tess) O'Shea, our inimitable prop from Cardiff, approached, limping appreciably.

Ian Smith solicitously enquired how the injury had happened. 'See 'ere, Ian,' said Tess. 'I was knackered from scrummaging, tired out from brilliant support-play and by the time I got the final pass from Keith Jarret I was almost buggered out. I only had yards to go to the try-line, so I swerved past the full-back like a gazelle and made the stupid mistake of side-stepping back into the bastard. I scored all right but I'm banjaxed now for a while. Too tired I was. Too good!'

Tess was far from depressed, always in good humour. I roomed with him often and was continually amused when he held up a photo of his then wife. 'I'm having such rotten bloody luck 'ere,' he'd say, looking at her picture, 'I'll have trouble getting off my mark, dearest, with you, when I get 'ome!' That was then; this was now.

ZERO POINT ONE SIX

FOURTEEN

There are None So Pure . . .

Many folks have assumed incorrectly that it is only with sober people that one can hold serious discussions. Curiously enough, meeting most of the really great people I've known occurred either during sporting activities, or when I happened to bump into them during mutual enjoyment of the bottle. I rarely met anybody abstemious then.

Almost all my friends take a drink nowadays, but that doesn't stop a drip-dried Doyle enjoying their company. The major differences now are that I don't drink, I probably meet them all less often, and I feel like asking myself on occasion, as my companions take more booze on board, 'Did I actually talk such unadulterated rubbish when I was drinking?' I know now that I did!

Even blokes whom I have always regarded as rocks of solid good sense suddenly begin to talk in parables after a few gargles! When I temporarily quit the jar in the early 1990s, this regularly amused and amazed me, and I often jokingly suggested that perhaps I should rejoin them in their merrymaking, to avoid missing out on all the *craic*.

Nowadays I don't give the demon firewater a second's thought. I think I have finally conquered my drinking

ZERO POINT ONE SIX

inclinations, and I am happily resigned never to touch it again. I have no ambitions either towards evangelism or to be a living proof of the reformed-whore syndrome. My halo is still the same size and at the similar rakish angle it was before; I don't want to polish it and I don't ever want to set myself up as a model to anybody. After all, I drank enough for two lifetimes.

However, deep down, I know that attraction to drink is a very dangerous drug which can take you over, like it did to me, exacting a terrible price both from loved ones and oneself. Unfortunately, you realise this only when it may be too late. However, I doubt if I would ever have become as involved in all that I had, certainly in rugby circles up to 1987, if I hadn't relished the camaraderie that the sport offered.

Nevertheless, it did set an unfortunate precedent for me, like eating a lot while you're still at the peak of your fitness as a player, and if you continue to do so after you've hung up your jockstrap, you're inclined to pile on the extra pounds quickly, particularly if you don't take preventative steps. That happened to me like a recurring decimal, especially from 1988 on.

On the other hand, the creeping paralysis of alcohol was incredibly difficult to shake off – far more difficult for me, in fact, than quitting smoking or the excess food and the hedonistic lifestyle. Life under the dependency of the drink felt as if I was threshing around helpless in a powerful tide – a sea which was welcoming much of the time, but was also rough and choppy, with malevolent humour and ominous intent.

I actually know very few thoroughbred blue-chip alcoholics. I was aware, of course, of the countless folk like me, who were fond of the gargle, even to excess at times, but addicts – no! Without in any way wishing to preach on the subject, I would like to suggest that if things are inclined to get out of hand in your life, or if the menacing merry-go-round beckons, then it is high time to confront your seducer head on before it is too late.

For me, the drink was extremely hard to pack in; for one thing it involved huge changes in my lifestyle – it entailed giving up a lot more than just drink: it meant eschewing male bonding, social gatherings and yarn-telling. All that stuff embraced the territory of the mind primarily, and unless the mind is prepared to make the painful, but very necessary changes, the body hasn't a hope of delivering on the physical side of things. A sudden massive stroke had made the decision for me, and the physical just followed along, obediently, like a dog on a lead. I was in no fit state to complain, anyway!

All the 'ifs', 'buts', 'ands' and 'would Is' do not matter a hoot now, and I won't try to give hypothetical answers to hypothetical questions, as my old friend Clive Rowlands from Swansea once replied at a press conference at Twickenham in 1986, when a Lions XV, of which we were both in charge, had just played a Rest of the World XV to celebrate the Rugby World's centenary.

The day before the game I had taken to heart Clive's admonition to 'turn the question around' if some reporters quizzed me. During an interview with a group of pleasant press guys, actually a 'no hassle' occasion, one bloke innocently asked, 'Ma, ma, Mick,' he said, 'is it ta ta ta ta true that you don't see eye to eye with Ja Ja Jacques Foroux?' (We had been joined by French players Serge Blanco, Jean Condom (or 'the other French second row', as Fred Cogley reputedly called him), Philippe Sella and Pierre Rodrigues for our second game against the Rest-of-the-World; Jacques, the French coach, had become my helper, interpreter and friend.)

Anyway, I looked the intrepid journalist right in the eye, and with Rowland's-backed bravado, I replied, amid pin-dropping silence, 'Dead right, Terry, I don't.'

'Whaaa wha why not?' he shot back, sensing a scandal.

'Because it's impossible to see eye-to-eye with a bloke who's only four foot nothing!' A cacophony of whoops drowned out further chat. Sad to say, I was only a wistful memory now, though.

The one saving grace, I suppose, was that I had been a happy drinker; drink never made me nasty or argumentative and never led me to strike anyone. But I now know, for certain, that it is worthwhile to seriously cut down your intake, if you are a regular boozer, plan your drinking arrangements as you would organise a household budget. *Of course* it is difficult, and awkward, but no matter how you cover up the true facts for someone else's benefit, you cannot fool yourself. Hindsight is never wrong; I had plenty of it. If I had my former life all over again, I hope I would have looked squarely at my problems. I hope I would have had the strength to confront them and the resolve to give up the booze. I wonder . . .

Total abstinence may have been the only way for people like me, and it may save *your* life, too, but it took a brain haemorrhage to save mine. I almost had to die to live again. Life's funny, isn't it?

———————————

Overeating, drinking *any* alcohol or entertaining any stress formed no part of the agenda in hospital. Getting better did. However, few things happen by chance; nothing worthwhile ever does. It took a lot of hard work. The cold turkey of the physical craving may have been camouflaged by the stroke, but subconsciously I must have cried in bitter mourning at the loss of a friend. I was still an invalid then, with a long journey in front of me. What temptations will come my way out in civvy street? I often wondered.

I had asked my physician, very soon after my escape to freedom, if I should ever drink again. 'In all seriousness, Mick,' said Eóin, 'I wouldn't if I were you; I don't know what it might do to your brain.'

'Well, doc,' said I, 'if *you* don't know, then I haven't a clue. I just won't drink.'

While I faced down the booze on my own with the 'help' of

a stroke, I realise that Alcoholics Anonymous may be the major solution for some people. It is after all a superb organisation and helps countless people all over the world. Thankfully, I was able to fly solo – so far anyway.

ZERO POINT ONE SIX

FIFTEEN

The New Reality

'Bygone images and scenes of early life have stolen my mind, like breezes blow from the spice-islands of Youth and Hope – those twin realities of this Phantom World.'

(Samuel Taylor Coleridge, *Table Talk*, 1835)

I left my *youth* behind me many years ago (even though I enjoyed every second of it) and take singular pleasure now in the countless fond memories of that purple period.

Hope, with luck, will be my companion until the day I die, and who knows what will happen in the next world? If we expired on Mars, or on the moon, then where would we go? I would naturally expect that there really is something other than just a scientific nothingness waiting for us when we finally relinquish our grip on mortality. I would hate to have lived my life in a *Phantom World*, a great void.

However, in direct contrast, a few days after waking up from my deep slumber, and meeting Mandy again, I felt her silently slipping the familiar gold band on my marriage finger; quietly, without fuss, not saying a word. It had conveyed a definite signal that she had fully accepted that I would now probably make it

and that we were a couple once more. She had obviously removed the ring as I lay in a coma.

Of all the things that could have motivated me most, that marriage ring was it. It made me feel loved and wanted and very definitely part of the future. Getting better was one thing, but the realisation of what Mandy had done gave me great hope. Obviously, stroke accentuates one's ambitions to get back to some semblance of normality; it heightens the senses. We all live in hope, so that any symbolism takes on a renewed importance.

Of major significance for me too was the thirtieth reunion of the 1968 touring British Lions' rugby team to South Africa, in Edinburgh's Dalmahoy Hotel, coinciding with the Scotland v South Africa match in November 1998.

In a nutshell, it was an unmitigated joy and a total therapy to meet again with all my old rugby mates, from each of the four countries, and all corners of the world now; and to recount stories and incidents from a naïve time thirty years earlier in an apartheid-riddled South Africa, when we thought we were the essence of sophistication!

There were two incidents from that unforgettable trip (Barry John often called it 'the last of the fun tours') that seem like they happened only yesterday. Bob Hiller, England's full-back and I were relaxing in our hotel lounge in Potchefstroom (why I don't know) when a brave woman journalist, looking for female-interest gossip, interviewed us. 'How did u find Sud Afrikka?' she asked, pencil at the ready.

'We turned right at Portugal!' said Hiller.

She didn't respond. 'How do u find Sud Afrikkan girls?' she asked.

'In public houses,' I offered, not to be outdone by the loquacious Londoner. Still no reaction from our female inquisitor.

'Which do u consider the best town in Sud Afrikka?'

'I reckon Salisbury,' [Rhodesia's Capital, now Harare] says Bob, as our erstwhile correspondent rode off in a blaze of dust.

The South African tourist board had commissioned Killarney Studios in Johannesburg to produce a short travelogue based loosely on the Lion's tour; the eager studio head sought out Roger Armeil from Edinburgh, Barry John from Cardiff and me to help with some zany shots throughout the tour – which we all gladly did, even becoming involved in the project by the end. We eagerly looked forward to reviewing all our handiwork in the finished article on the last week.

The three budding Sean Connerys waited in our hotel lobby when the studio bloke phoned to break the news that a fire had destroyed the studios overnight – and the video tape of all three of us in full frontal action also went up in smoke. What a waste of incredible talent. Posterity is probably grateful!

All the events of one's youth, and of the recent past as an adult, may suddenly assume a much greater significance, particularly while one is in the very eye of the struggle. In addition to my efforts towards rehabilitation, the love, attention and care that I received had a huge bearing on my recovery. I probably didn't fully appreciate it then but I certainly know it now. When you reflect on the plight of severely afflicted people, is it not wholly unacceptable that so many should find themselves shunned by everybody of any authority, except for their immediate families, as a burden to progress? I know, for sure, from organisations like the Volunteer Stroke Scheme and Headway Ireland that many unfortunates are thrown out of hospitals, to be abandoned as if from a dumper truck on to a society that cannot really cater for their more demanding welfare. Just as certain as we do not appear to have the facilities to handle the special needs of 'difficult' young people, our *great* and *good* welfare system fails the most vulnerable among us. It is as if the actual conditions that they live in would mess up any favourable statistics being waved around by our photo-opportunistic political leaders.

Surely society has no right imposing its own amnesia on its less fortunate members, turning its physical and mental back on them at their time of real-life crisis. Is it not pointless for our medical authority luminaries to be waxing eloquent about scientific breakthroughs, health initiatives and the latest finding of medical research, often in a strangely silent vacuum, while seemingly ignoring what is happening in our hospitals every single day?

The thalidomide scandal of the late 1960s should have taught us to be more questioning about extrapolating 'research' findings in animals and their application to human beings. The missing digits, horrifically distorted and abbreviated limbs were nature's testament that the sedative effects anticipated in pregnant women did not translate from female rats. It had caused thousands of birth defects world-wide before being implicated with certainty; it is now feared that the sad condition will project into following generations.

I trained to become a vet, and my role, that for which I recited with all fervour the Hippocratic Oath when I was conferred with my degree, was to make a solemn promise to preserve life, not to destroy it in the name of science. If medical progress demands that we should ignore our basic instincts, I'm sorry for it, and all I can say is to hell with all such progress. As such, it is only a further development in organised barbarity; all in the quasi-advancement of science. Of course it now strikes me that prevention is far and away the best option – unless you have a death wish – and far, far surer.

Progress may appreciably increase the survival rate of some people from brain haemorrhage and other life-threatening conditions, but that still would leave a huge swathe of normal people who could die prematurely and needlessly. Just imagine the desolation that this causes, and already happens on a daily basis. It hardly bears thinking about. If I had died, I wouldn't have had time even to make my farewells to the people who mean a lot to me. I would never again, in this life anyway, see them, nor our dogs and ponies. They are my friends, too. I would be missing out on so much that matters to me, exchanging it for the dubious pleasures of the after-life. No thanks; not just yet!

Had I snuffed it, it would have been nobody's fault but mine. It's basically because I was stupid and wasteful with my life and talents, allowing overindulgence to creep up steadily like ivy on a tree, and become the norm. It is opportune now, though, to emphasise that love and living are too important to me, that I have a long road in front of me yet, and that when I finally quit this life I want to be very old, fully satisfied with my lot and ready to go to meet my maker.

While my grown-up children, Andrew, Sharon and Amanda, are incredibly important to me, and while Emma, at twelve, will need a lot of help and support for a long time yet, Mandy is my life; they all have their own careers to look forward to, but I owe my continued hold on this world to her most of all. 'For richer, for poorer, in sickness and in health' had taken on real meaning for us; they weren't just pious words anymore.

And so, I must say that whatever you might think of doing yourself, that is anything within reason, of course, I have already drunk it, eaten it, smoked it or 'lived' it. I have earned a roomful of gold medals for excess. At the finishing line of all this madness, I can tell you, friends, 'It was not worth the effort.' No way; I missed out on too much. I was blind *and* daft. Youth led me into trouble, but hope helped me survive, to fight other battles.

SIXTEEN

Mandy's Story

DURING

The Intensive Care Unit had bright fluorescent lighting, various monitors bleeping and flashing different colours, phones frequently ringing and people rushing about; small wonder that Mick was hallucinating. He thrashed about the narrow bed, a big bear of a man reduced to a tangle of tubes and confusion.

Ever the entertainer, Mick injected the occasional dose of black humour when he tried to answer the phone, hold business meetings or order another round of drinks for everyone and their friends, not to mention demanding to pay the bill and move to a hotel with better service! This was counter-balanced by the pain of watching my beloved husband in severe discomfort – repeatedly ripping out his nasal tube and other drips, so that they needed to be reinserted until he was bruised and raw, struggling and fighting, despite the two holes and drainage tube at the base of his skull, his betrayed face dripping with sweat and his badly infected lungs gasping for every suffocatingly elusive breath. In this fashion the minutes merged into hours into days. Fleeting recognition and slight rays of hope were interspersed with urgent intervention and further heart-stopping crises.

Life in the waiting room just outside the Intensive Care Unit was like another world: family members waited and prayed, sometimes sobbing as loved ones breathed and then didn't, responded and then didn't, recognised and then didn't, came around or died – leaving a gaping, threatening space where the wheeled bed had been until the next 'case' and the next worried, white-faced relatives filled the gap.

Laughter here was as inappropriate as at a funeral. If a patient rallied, all joined in the relief as hope-filled calls were hastily made from the payphone outside the door. We shared some sort of bond – like plane-crash survivors, we were all in this together. We shared and traded holy relics, reverently placing them on our unresponsive loved ones and fervently repeating our desperate prayers.

Some patients were old and weary, wending a difficult path towards eternity; some like Mick were ruddy-faced *bon viveurs*, somewhat indignant at being told 'Time, gentlemen, please.' Others were mere children, teenage sports stars giving shocking significance to the injury statistics. All were now in the hands of God.

BEFORE

'Desperado'

Let's just say I didn't marry Mick for his waistline! Somewhere inside this fuzzy outline there was the spirit of a taut, fit athlete – he had the broad shoulders and narrow hips and strong, well-muscled legs but the rest 'needed work'. Like many retired rugby stars, he had gone to seed a little.

Of course I thought I would change all that. By the time I realised that the only one who could change Mick was himself, I had fallen in love with him and could only hope and pray that with gentle encouragement and lots of rebuilding of his self-esteem he could learn to love himself enough to alter his destructive lifestyle.

When I cooked healthy, low-fat dinners Mick would often fail to show up, preferring to spend the evening in a pub followed by a large Chinese meal with like-minded 'partners in crime'. After many evenings at home with our baby, frantic that he might have driven into some ditch, wanting to call the police but afraid of him losing his license (looking back perhaps that may have been just the sort of 'kick' he needed), I simply gave up worrying – I could no longer stand the pressure of waiting for a heart-attack, or worse. I went into a form of denial – concentrating on our child (mentally vowing not to have another baby in this less than idyllic set-up), our animals, and keeping my own body and soul together.

I missed the real Mick, who was so wonderful and beloved. I often felt lonely and cheated – if he loved Emma and me how could he let himself go like this? At the time I did not understand the compulsions of an alcoholic and that his seemingly selfish behaviour was not caused by a lack of love. Many so-called 'friends' and others are always ready to encourage excessive drinking; if only they could see the resulting pain.

'For better or for worse' – this was for worse. I prayed to God that my husband would stop drinking and shed his massive weight to fulfil his potential as the man I still hoped (hope, though, at this time was fading) was in there somewhere.

EMMA

The day of Mick's brain bleed, our daughter Emma, then seven years old, was suffering from gastro-enteritis. I felt torn and frantic seeing her white frightened little face trying so hard to be brave as I had to leave her with my mother, Sonia, so I could speed after the ambulance to Beaumont Hospital.

Later on when Mick came out of Intensive Care, Emma would come to the hospital for the day with me, and would spend hours quietly drawing and colouring beautiful pictures to brighten up the walls of her daddy's sick room. When she should have been at the seaside on those beautiful hot summer days, instead she inhabited the mini-city of the large hospital, speaking in hushed whispers and unavoidably picking up on the seriousness of the situation. As Mick slowly recovered, enough to leave his room in a wheelchair and get out into the hospital grounds, we gratefully breathed in the fresh air and the rather dusty beauty of the few trees, bedding plants and shrubs in the litter-strewn garden.

As we finally could allow ourselves to believe that he was going to live (a definite miracle – all praise and thanks to God!), I was anxious to get him home and nurse him back to health. I was so innocent. I thought I was taking home a gentle invalid whom I could spoil, pamper and care for, but no one bothered to let me, his next of kin, know about the personality changes, the mood swings and frustration that frequently occur in the aftermath of brain trauma.

The person I brought home was an angry, petulant stranger. Totally dependent and vulnerable, yet also unpredictable and always ready with a lethal verbal missile to hurt and invalidate the opinions of those closest to him, as well as the occasional unfortunate stranger who happened to cross paths with a wounded, damaged man, locked in his own painful, personal struggle back to life.

My new prayer was, please, God, help me to love this man. I was so very tired and lonely. We went into survival mode. I neglected and avoided dear friends, fearing that a kind word could sweep away my shaky countenance that everything was now wonderful and fine; it wasn't fine and I knew that with all my responsibilities I could not afford to let the floodgates open. Did people really die of sadness?

Eventually, one dark evening, I almost cracked, as my very best efforts to appease this new husband had once more failed miserably. I could see no light at the end of the tunnel, for no medic or social worker had ever explained that Mick's mood swings could eventually improve. I left the house, got into my jeep, alone, without Emma, my greatest treasure, and drove away. I wanted to disappear, to get off this rollercoaster and never return.

I did come back later that night. No one had missed me, but I had frightened myself and I knew I must get help. My GP diagnosed depression (a common condition in both carers without adequate support or respite as well as in the cared-for – hindsight is so illuminating!) and prescribed a popular drug to help me cope. In my heart I knew that rather than a chemical imbalance I was suffering from emotional and physical exhaustion and needed a holiday, but I was glad to grasp this chemical crutch. Instead of relief, I experienced side effects so severe that I collapsed, barely able to swallow water. My wonderfully kind mother came over and I did get a couple of days in bed. Her concern about me helped to give me renewed strength to carry on, albeit now with the added sense of hopelessness that even a 'happy pill' could not help me to escape.

An angel in the form of a good friend, Daphne, counselled me and helped me to realise that I did have a reason to feel bad. I was mourning for the loss of my husband as he had been, as well as watching many of our hopes and dreams fade away. As a family, our futures were changed and now tinged with insecurity. Our young daughter was living through experiences no child should have to cope with. I missed the laughter and fun and happy safe feeling at home.

Sometimes I tried to overcompensate Emma for the state we found ourselves in and for the differences between her father and those of her friends, but she was always a wonderful blessing to have and seeing her sense of humour, not to mention her sharp intellect, and acute sense of justice – traits inherited from Mick – frequently helped to give a glimmer of the real man I had loved.

One way of coping with Mick's grumpiness was to try and make a joke of his ill-humour and irrational outbursts by inventing rude names for him – we could defuse the moment with a glance at each other; although it was often difficult to differentiate between the man we loved and the behaviour we dreaded.

AFTERMATH

It's now over five years since the brain bleed. Mick is still a little wobbly on his feet at times, particularly if he is very tired or stressed. He is gradually losing weight and often looks so well that I can almost forget to worry about him!

An old friend told me that when he had been gravely ill he had said some things to one of his daughters, and, despite knowing that he was unaware at the time, he felt that she has never quite forgiven or trusted him again. Of course I understand how she feels, but time – lots of it – does help and heal.

I am filled with respect for Mick's bravery and fortitude in never giving up, in continuing to work every available hour to keep 'food on the table' – often when he felt dreadful; many lesser mortals would have simply thrown in the towel.

His resolve in completely giving up alcohol (and chocolate!) seems miraculous, not to mention his efforts to control his temper. Much of his gentleness and a large amount of his confidence have returned, obviously helping his relationship with Emma. He remains one of the most intelligent men I have met.

Sometimes God moves in mysterious ways. I believe that perhaps Mick was such a hard case that he needed a dramatic rebirth! Like many labours, it was long and difficult, but the new improved man may well prove it was all worth it.

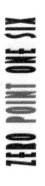

A FEW WORDS ABOUT HOSPITALS . . .

Of course there are many wonderful people in hospitals – angels who literally pull vulnerable and ill patients through. Human nature being what it is though, there are also some who should really choose a different career.

A little gentleness and the preservation of a patient's dignity should be obvious – sadly this is not always the case. For example, one morning I arrived to find my husband, recovering from brain surgery, with a new bloody gash on his forehead. Just off the feeding tube, he had been administered a laxative. When he later rang his bell (with extreme difficulty), it was unanswered, forcing Mick, who was not able to walk, to try and crawl to the toilet. Naturally he crashed to the floor and lay there until he was found, bruised and degraded. When I enquired as to what had happened, I discovered this type of incident was treated as routine.

The brilliance, humanity and kindness of some of the overworked doctors, surgeons and consultants at the hospital served to highlight the sheer arrogance of other members of staff; this arrogance affected their dealings with patients and their carers and families.

THE THERAPEUTIC EFFECTS OF ANIMALS . . .

Little
While Mick was still incarcerated in Beaumont Hospital, and as soon as our wheelchair excursions extended as far as the main entrance hall, Emma and I brought two of our little dogs, Daisy and Bunty, to visit him.

Although slightly unnerved by the noise and smells of a busy hospital, Bunty sat up on her little rounded bottom and waved her front paws and smiled endearingly at him, irresistibly bringing a responsive smile to Mick's strained countenance.

Daisy, Mick's self-appointed nurse and protector, sat up on his knee and tenderly and delicately licked his sore, semi-sightless eyes. When it was time to return the dogs to the car Daisy pulled back on her lead, worried and reluctant to leave her beloved master.

Eventually, when Mick came home for an afternoon, then a day and then a night, Daisy never let him out of her sight. She immediately found his wound, still painful and raw, having become seriously infected in hospital, and gently cleaned it with her tongue – undoubtedly helping it to finally heal up. She became Mick's constant companion, always curled up next to him on the bed or squeezed quietly beside him in the armchair, never taking offence if he was having a bad day, faithful to the last. Daisy, a quaint, hairy little terrier with bushy eyebrows, who came to us as an unwanted stray, an exhausted, rejected wee creature with a heart still full of love and her tiny generous spirit bringing incalculable curative powers to her adoptive family.

Large

Approximately one and a half years into Mick's long, slow recovery, I needed something extra in my life to keep me sane. Some people take up golf or embark on extra-marital affairs; I drove westwards one blustery day and found a highly sensitive Anglo-Arab bay mare, four years old. I named her Amber Light and she certainly became the light of my life.

A spirited, nervous, flighty handful to begin with – we had to learn to trust each other and she encouraged me to begin a study of 'alternative' methods of horseriding. She is maturing into a highly intelligent and gentle friend, still with the occasional frisson of excitability just to keep life interesting and challenging! Even just watching Amber playing with our other ponies, delicate Araby nostrils flared, head and tail high and proud, her beautiful action prancing and dancing along, makes my heart soar. This may seem over the top to some – but any true horse lover will understand!

If this appears to digress from the business of Mick's story, I include it to illustrate the extreme importance of an outside interest or safety valve for carers. It may help keep them going through the bad times, and animals, with their forgiving and giving natures, together with the inevitable encounters with other people who you meet while caring for them or exercising them, can provide a significant lifeline in times of loneliness and isolation. They ask for so little in return and deserve to be treated with respect and dignity as befits any vulnerable species entrusted into our care by God.

ZERO POINT ONE SIX

SEVENTEEN

And in the Meantime . . .

I have been truly delighted by the steady progress I've been making; five years on, the hard struggle and the often apparently futile efforts towards recovery have finally fulfilled my overriding desire to get better.

Happily I interact more easily nowadays and I have found that stress does not figure so largely in my lifestyle anymore – I've either learned to handle it better or else to simply ignore it. Close relationships with members of my family continue to be excellent; recently celebrating my sixtieth birthday with my wife and four children in Wexford was an occasion of incredible fun for me. I felt truly blessed and unsixty-like!

My balance is almost normal and will probably always remain slightly compromised; but few people other than myself would notice. I've relearned to ride a bicycle since July 2000, and after a few initial bouts of wobbly progress I was soon enjoying pedal-power again – a long, long way from the meandering wheelchair.

In October 2000 I joined Naas Health and Fitness Club with Mandy; me becoming an athlete again, much to our genuine amazement! However, slowly but purposefully I am making reasonable progress at this fitness lark. Even though I always had

the ambition to become a gym-floor Lothario, often well hidden, I somehow never envisaged reaching that seemingly unattainable state after my stroke.

Unbelievably I am now trying to atone, with the urgency of a reckless turtle, for all those years I studiously ignored treadmills and circuits, exercise bikes and the rest of gymworld's paraphernalia. Of course it is wholly different from the early struggles in the gymnasium of the Rehabilitation Hospital: I can now gaze with amazement and a certain gratification (that I can use much of it) at the health centre's fitness equipment; even daring to picture myself a physically fit specimen once again. The progression from the exercises of recovery to the training regimen for athletic fitness is really huge and now seems incredible in just over five years.

Daily events like showering, shaving, dressing, driving and walking have assumed a large degree of normality, but are never humdrum. I'll take nothing for granted again. I am continually reminded by the extent of the many improvements I have made in such a short while; the difficult chores of a year or so ago are now commonplace.

I stopped corresponding on rugby and other sports about three years ago, but I've begun giving talks to various groups again, as before, on motivation, team-building, agenda-setting and focusing – everything seems to be that much clearer now; and again I love talking to my friends at Rugby Club dinners, as if I had never been away.

My regular visits to Eóin O'Brien and Conor Devine have changed from quarterly to once annually; they variously check my weight, blood pressure and heart function. I am a familiar 'post-graduate' figure in Beaumont in the Haematology Department, having my blood sampled and analysed for various elements. In addition Professor O'Brien decreed initially that I should have a regular 24-hour blood-pressure monitor fitted to my arm. These were all within normal limits and I now go once a year to be checked over; a lot less regularly than even before my stroke.

I realise of course that I was luckier than many people with stroke, but the whole process has certainly proved conclusively that fairly dramatic gains in one's former capabilities can be made by almost anyone sufficiently determined. During all my rugby coaching days I always let players know that I would never blame any bloke for trying out something unusual or extra bold; instead I would almost certainly hold the other fourteen players, who failed to support him, responsible for any failure. Only thus could the shackles of conservatism and uniformity be consigned to the Kleenex waste basket.

There is little doubt that if the efforts of rehabilitating patients are brave and determined enough, and if they are fully supported by family and friends, success is far more predictable; for 'no man is an island', nor woman either. Unfortunately there are no guarantees, just predictions.

Naturally I realise that some less fortunate people will only recover incompletely from their injuries; that may be sad, but nevertheless undeniable. In my relatively short experience a consistent mistake many people make is to shut out their loved ones as they begin to withdraw from any real-life, close involvement. Such patients often tell their heartbroken loved ones to forget them, find someone new and make new lives for themselves, as they themselves give up on life as they had known it.

Painful it most certainly is for both parties, and wholly unnecessary, even unrealistic. I also know that in some instances head-injured people do actually mean what they say. I am certain that though some may utter unkind words of dismissal to close relatives, deep down many don't mean it; they are just seeking the reassurance that they are truly wanted. This often takes a long time to resolve, but is well worth the effort.

Without in any way indulging in deep psychological analysis, I would say that I fully understand how miserable both parties may feel; I can assure patients that what their carers wish for *most of all* is to become thoroughly involved, to help with repair and

181

recovery and to plan the future together, to stay with them. That is an incredible start.

In all instances that I know of I feel sure that the hiccough of stroke or head injury is only just that to the nearest and dearest. If my advice is ever sought, I can honestly say, 'Hang in there, be patient, your other half does not mean it, and things will come round in the end. It certainly won't be like before, but who knows it may even be better! I was a stupid, awkward bugger, too, you know.'

As circumstances have permitted all three of us to return to Lanzarote this spring for the first time since 1994, its magic was more focused, if anything.

How did I feel? I had been curious about the four-hour plane trip, but it was hitch-free. The overriding feeling I suppose was 'I thought I'd never see this place again'; and I continually pinched myself to help me realise how lucky I was.

Everything was the same, except for the logical progress of seven years, but it felt, smelt, tasted and looked even better than before, to my definitely biased eyes. Mandy, Emma and I got on famously, no more 'wick bothering', and my eyesight, balance, speech and fitness, in fact everything about life for me, felt even better than previously.

I walked most mornings, often up to eight miles, swam many days, ate and shopped and talked to loads of people, drove for about half a day (enough believe me) and generally did anything I had done before, except jog. I know now at last that I will never aspire to be a poolside toyboy, but I had one hell of a holiday!

Two incidents impacted on the trip; first, the untimely death from cancer of all in rugby's friend, Gordon Brown, made me grieve for him and sadly remember the good times. Second, the escalating progress of Foot and Mouth disease in Britain made me rail at the apparently puny efforts, wholly inconsequential, that were taken early on in the course of this scourge, by the British Ministry of Agriculture. It appeared as if they'd given the two-fingered salute to Britain's farmers, wholly mis-understanding the nature and consequence of the disease. Pity!

Still, I must admit that a brain haemorrhage was one holiday break that I would not recommend to anyone. Naturally, I am sorry now that 'I used my youth as if it were a wand', but I did.

I was able to venture out to mow the lawn last Easter holiday, rescuing the four-wheeled, electric-engined question mark from its winter hibernation; I had fully expected to be assailed by a similar unsteadiness and the pain of instability that I experienced while cutting that grass last autumn. Incredibly, almost miraculously in fact, the unsteadinesss had all evaporated like the rains and cold winds of winter and early spring. The 'healing hands of time' had shown their worth, producing by themselves another giant step on the road to recovery. Anyway, it appears so. I was thrilled, although it seems such a small, inconsequential thing to be happy about!

ZERO POINT ONE SIX

EPILOGUE

The Future is a Crystal Ball

Osmosis is a familiar term in chemistry; it describes the passing of a solvent through a semi-permeable membrane into a more concentrated solution on the other side. Both concentrations then become equal. What has happened to my life in many ways resembles a type of *osmosis in reverse*, in that my core being, the entity that is the real essence of me, left my body like a solvent, passed through the semi-permeable membrane of a brain haemorrhage, on the other side of which there was a debatable *nothingness*, and emerged, *scathed*, on the other side of that two-way mirror. I was naturally a very different person to the one left behind, but that central part of me, the defining spirit, the soul, stayed intact.

The concentrations (or outward appearances) may have ended up similar on either side, but the ingredients that made up the new solution that was me were completely different; and they certainly needed to be, for I didn't want to go through that saga again. It was as if I had been dumped, soiled and exhausted, into a washing machine, put through a tumble drier set permanently at spin, coming out the far end cleansed. As well as that, I felt emptied of all previous, irrelevant thoughts and weaned off bad tendencies in relation to booze, food, stress and wayward living; I was ready to face most things.

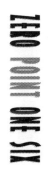

It felt almost if I had become increasingly human, as more and more people demonstrated their support. Probably it was there all the time, only I didn't think enough about it, or appreciate it.

I have often been asked, 'Will it happen again?' I don't honestly know, but I hope not. The only guarantee worth anything in this life, the absolute certainty, is death, but I'm not ready for that just yet. Life is much too exciting to experience and savour all the things about the new me in the days and years that I hope stretch ahead. I would simply hate it, having gone through so much over the past few years, dragging myself towards the beaches of normality, or as near as possible, for me to kick the bucket prematurely.

What kinds of feelings, you might ask, dominate my conscious hours now? Well, primarily there is incredible gratitude for being one of the zero point one six per cent, for having been spared and being able to make up in some way for my previous omissions. I know I'll fall down here and there along the way, but I shall try that bit harder.

I will also be forever beholden to my close family, friends and associates for showing me that I *do* count, that they care for me, in some cases intensely, and want me around for a good while longer. But there's too much leeway to make up; even if I lived for a couple of lifetimes, I couldn't make amends for all my past transgressions, and so I won't even try; but I *do* regret them deeply.

I never fully realised before just how crucial one's faculties are – the ability to express one's feelings, to converse, to walk, cycle, drive and all the countless, incidental little things (which normal society takes for granted); these have now assumed a central relevance. In fact, they have become overwhelmingly important, and, with rather more emphasis, are now part and parcel of being a living human being again.

I feel damaged all right and probably slightly flawed; there are a few things I can't do now that I did before. On the opposite side of the equation, I am far brighter and more relaxed nowadays and I can take my time doing things that I didn't bother much about before my brain haemorrhage.

It had never occurred to me what it would be like to be so dependent on other people. It has put a whole new, broader perspective on life for me now. My heart goes out to all dependants and their families; I hope they preserve their fighting spirit and the motivation to keep struggling on against the odds, not giving up, always aiming for their own personal goals. Often progress feels like three steps backward for every one forward, but like the tortoise we can get there in the end, in our own good time.

The brain haemorrhage taught me many lessons. It has pinpointed how of such little consequence other people's ambitions and agendas are to my own life now; it has highlighted unequivocally that the Joneses are not worth keeping up with anyway. Personally, I have always commiserated with them on their need to be perfect.

I am fascinated by the human spirit and astounded by the ability of the body to repair, and the mind to heal itself. If you should ever contemplate the spider's web, which it has woven with such loving care and ingenuity, you might observe some interesting things: as the spider lies ready to pounce, you can clearly see the busy arachnid patiently repairing any tears or breaks in its silky maze – time after time, in no hurry, like fishermen mending their nets. It brings home so strikingly, that even something so perfect and wondrous can be damaged too, and in need of reconstruction.

In the end that simple spider was the role model for me – an object of surprise and inspiration, as it stoically accepts life's setbacks, and quietly and purposefully goes about putting everything back in working order again, even though it had become seriously damaged. It never shows impatience or rage;

just quiet determination. That's what a subarachnoid haemorrhage, a stroke, does to you: it stimulates you to swim towards recovery. Although you might feel feeble at first, your progress becomes more confident as you strike out for the far shore of the pothole.

Overindulgence of almost everything was my problem. Life was good then – a lovely mirage; I had enough natural ecstasy without taking any of the manufactured stuff. But I don't judge anybody now. How could I? I have no right to.

I have also learned, to my cost, that prevention is very definitely better than cure and far, far less costly on everyone. But I'm lucky; I'm alive to do more than just tell the tale and I am thankful to all sorts of people and to God for that. There *is* hope for everybody; depression and demotivation may be the usual consequences of stroke, but they must be confronted and dismissed by you, yourself, and they can be. You may get a lot of help from others, but in the end it is all down to yourself; there are no magic tablets to make mind-matters go away. Self-help continues to be the only way.

Eleanor Roosevelt was right: 'People can only make you feel inferior if you let them.' In the end the future is all that lies ahead; the past, with luck, will not come back to haunt us. It is a very personal future and one which probably occupies my mind more nowadays.

As we are left to sort out our private thoughts and clamber on top of our new worries, we come to really appreciate that 'There is little point in setting your sails if you don't know where you're going.'

Finally, though I haven't met him since, I must thank the guy who drank pints of Guinness in Mulvey's pub long ago. He was the bloke driving me in the ambulance on the way to Beaumont Hospital from Naas on that momentous Sunday, 14 July 1996, when I nearly woke up dead. Thanks is also due to the surgeon who happened to be in Beaumont on that Sunday and saved my life. Thanks to them and many others I can now look forward to my future and learn from the past. But hope is like a smouldering fire; it often needs to be vigorously fanned before it bursts into flame – and ambitions will follow and turn themselves into reality. Life's like that.

Look after yourselves. You owe yourselves that, at least, for only fools fail.

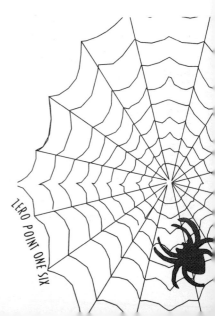